You can be an

EXPERT PRESCRIBER

*The MASTER KEY to all locking
situations in prescribing*

Dr. Rashmin Deshmukh

BHMS

B. JAIN PUBLISHERS (P) LTD.

AN ISO 9001 : 2000 CERTIFIED COMPANY

HOW TO BE AN EXPERT PRESCRIBER

Edition: 2006

Price: Rs. 99.00

Published by Kuldeep Jain for

B. Jain Publishers (P) Ltd.

1921, Street No. 10, Chuna Mandi,
Paharganj, New Delhi 110 055 (INDIA)
Phones: 91-11-2358 0800, 2358 1100, 2358 1300, 2358 3100
Fax: 91-11-2358 0471; *Email:* bjain@vsnl.com
Website: **www.bjainbooks.com**

Printed in India by
J.J. Offset Printers
522, FIE, Patpar Ganj, Delhi - 110 092

ISBN : 81-8056-675-7
BOOK CODE : BD-5904

Dedication
In Memory of My 'ATYA'
Late Smt. KAMALTAI JOSHI
and
Once again to
Dr. S. KARNAD
My revered teacher and a dedicated
Hahnemannian Homeopath

PREFACE

I considered homeopathy my cup of tea until I was studying it as a science, but soon when it came to the actual application of the laws of this spectacular science, I realized that it was definitely my cup of tea but a cup filled upto the brim with unheard difficulties and unforeseen obstacles. There were 'N' number of practical problems and umpteen difficulties encountered by me in medical practice and each one needed a right solution, indeed a perfectly practical one. Theoretical guidelines could but just do little to pull a physician like me out of these difficulties. There were innumerable books that told you 'How to study?' 'What to prescribe?' even 'What not to do?' but they were of a limited help.

I needed a book that could tell me 'Just how to do it!' I delved for information into books. Most of them failed to cover the very basic, practical, unforeseen, 'sure to emerge' problems. They were away from the 'ground realities' that a physician had to face while battling with the disease. There were books, which hardly considered a 'prescribing situation' a physician was into and were written giving sole consideration to ideal situations of prescribing. In reality there were many situations in which a homeopathic physician landed, where his hands were tied due to various considerations, limitations, possibilities and perils. There were many limitations of the law of cure and of the doctrines of the science. The cooperation from the patients as regards to the observation and expression of the disease peculiarities was most of the times disappointing. Most of the patients not being fully aware about homeopathy as a science could not furnish the information relevant to a physician in making a scientific homeopathic prescription.

I felt having been pushed into a battleground where I had to fight against the ever so powerful diseases in a very limited arena, with the dynamic weapons, which could be used under limitations and amidst multiple restrictions. Soon I realized, how difficult it was to obey homeopathic principles and to employ a therapeutic method scientifically in order to affect a cure even in the simplest deviations in the state of health. As a student of homeopathy I was a believer at core but in the primary phase of my medical practice my 'roots of belief' seemed to loose their grip in the sacred soil of homeopathy. But somewhere the roots had to be again strongly fixed.

I felt that a very distinct, more so a practical approach had to be critically employed in order to overcome all these difficulties. So in a valiant attempt to fight with the difficulties and diseases I went ahead under the guidance of some books and teachings of my revered teacher Dr. S. Karnad and I started artistically applying the scientific method my teacher taught me. Certain things established as the norms and 'essentials' of my prescribing, which when implemented yielded me nothing but Hahnemannian Cure. This practical application of a standardized approach, lead to the belief in me that one could master homeopathic prescribing.

I must mention that only Homeopathic Philosophy came to my respite in all the trying times and strong principles always made me stand firm where the disease seemed to be more powerful and difficulties dominating. My further experiences coupled with the practical application of the doctrines hepled me to develop an art of prescribing and took me to the shore of some wonderful cures only to multiply my faith in the science by infinity. I was astonished, overwhelmed and infact dumbfound to find how a 'practical approach and attitude' based on doctrines could work wonders towards achieving a cure. It could really make things simple and simply excellent.

Soon I held a belief contrary to the popular one that one cannot master homeopathic prescribing. I discovered it was 'easier done than said' but it was important to come down to earth and many things needed to be located and attended and a method skillfully applied, verified and ultimately mastered. You needed to develop your own art. It is possible for us to master the techniques of prescribing if not the science in totality. You need to train yourself as a homeopathic technician to be an accomplished prescriber. One could never conquer knowledge for its vastness a technique for sure could be mastered. I strongly believe that one can definitely be an expert, a professionally trained artist (with a self imparted training) in the art of prescribing on the logical base of the science and thus a MASTER PRESCRIBER. You just need to have a knack of it which is cleverness acquired through practice enabling to do so skillfully. And this is what the book is all about.

The practical guidelines incorporated in the book are easily adaptable, simple to implement and fully in accordance with the homeopathic philosophy. This book will be certainly of immeasurable value in prescribing to students exposed to numerous cases at college hospitals, to the interns standing on the first step of their prescribing ladders to CURE, and the physicians who even after being trained by most experienced hands still feel the ridge between theory and practice. It will for sure enhance their prescribing skills. The work will serve as an aid in prescribing at all levels. Something that will provide a master key, to all the 'locking situations' in practice.

The book will also be very useful to amateur prescriber and people who read and venture into 'homeopathy at home.' It will not only help people interested in study and practice of homeopathy learn and develop a right approach to its study and practice, but also contribute in cultivating a scientific attitude towards homeopathy.

Gaining mastery in homeopathic prescribing should never be seen as a special achievement but it is a need of a science so deep, detailed and critical. Mastery should only be a basic requirement so that the science is rightly and successfully practiced. Further sections will elaborate the need for the mastery.

My previous work, which guided how to study and approach homeopathy as a science in totality and various homeopathic subjects in particular took birth when I had just completed my study in homeopathy and realized the numerous difficulties faced by the students in the study of homeopathy. I was heavily burdened at conscience to come up with a work, which could further guide a novice in ' How to do it'—how to implement and execute what had been studied so systematically. This book is something I owe to this moral obligation.

From the author's eyes I see it as a work that could guide a novice in his medical practice right from the word 'Go' and also instill a scientific spirit, in the light of homeopathic philosophy. All the guidelines in the book are based on the principles and values, which my revered teacher Dr. S. Karnad incorporated in me and I credit it all to him. This book is an expression of my experience of application of a scientific method more efficiently and effectively. It is a reflection of the pearls of knowledge I gathered from my teacher.

The work is practical yet logical, encompassing a very down to earth, yet a scientific approach to homeopathic prescribing. One may look at this book as a literary extension of sky scraping spirits of a young homeopathic heart. It won't be wrong to interpret so, surely the spirits that went into the book were as high as that, but one needs to believe the feet were always fixed to the strong ground of homeopathic principles, and shall be so forever.

January 2006
Nagpur, India   **Dr. Rashmin Deshmukh**

ABOUT THE AUTHOR

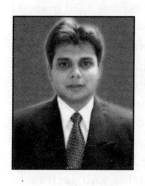 The author, Dr. Rashmin Deshmukh, was born on 16th December, 1976 at New Delhi. His mother Mrs. Radhika Deshmukh and father Mr. G. G. Deshmukh both were interested in homeopathy. Thus being born in the type of the environment that was conducive to homeopathy he had a natural inclination towards it. Highly influenced by the science he outrightly decided to undertake the study of homeopathy. He completed his degree in homeopathy from Nagpur University in 1999. He had a brilliant academic career and twice secured second meritorious position in Nagpur University.

He received the *Hahnemann Paritoshik 1999* instituted by the Homeopathic Medical Association of India and Homeopaths Association Chandrapur for his academic excellence. He was lecturer in anatomy for some time in the same college where he studied. He then had the fortune of studying under the able guidance of Dr. S. Karnad, an erudite person, a physician of unique qualities of Nagpur. Later he started his private practice in Nagpur. Besides, he is also a prolific writer and has to his credit many articles on varied subjects, which have been published in national-dailies.

He has authored two books on homeopathy one titled *Homeopathy As a Career,* a very useful book for students as well as physicians, and another *Baddhakosstatta (Constipation) Ani Homeopathy* which highlights the effectiveness of homeopathic treatment in constipation. He has also written a book of short stories titled *Days of Life* based on his life during youth. He has been engaged in social activities and renders his honorary services to an old people's home and an orphanage in Nagpur. He gives free consultation for de-addiction at his clinic in Nagpur. He is the Honorary Treasurer, Homeopathic Study Circle(HSC) Nagpur and Chief Adviser to Orange City Homeopath Association(OCHA). He is a strong advocator and propagator of scientific homeopathy (homeopathy practiced in accordance to the philosophy.) He has been rigorously chasing the cause by writing articles and letters in newspapers and by delivering lectures and talks at various places.

This book is his long thoughtout venture sincerely intended to spread the light of scientific homeopathy amongst youth and veterans.

FOREWORD

To create a scientific awareness rather we can say a scientific approach amongst homeopaths, this book "You Can Be An Expert Prescriber — The Master Key to all Locking Situations in Prescribing" by Dr. Rashmin Deshmukh is a brilliant attempt.

Not only a dream but it should also be the aim of every physician to become an expert prescriber. The practical guidelines incorporated in the book are easy to understand and are easily adaptable. They are simple to implement and are fully in accordance with the homeopathic philosophy. To develop a right approach towards prescribing and cultivating a scientific attitude towards homeopathy is a successful attempt by the author in the right direction.

Dr. Mridula Pandey

Sr. M.O., Govt. of Delhi

CONTENTS

CHAPTER I

AN EXPERTISE IN PRESCRIBING

HISTORY OF HOMEOPATHIC PRESCRIBING

Dr. Samuel Hahnemann introduced the system of homeopathy in the year 1790 through his essay, 'An Essay on the New Principle for Ascertaining The Curative Powers of Drugs and some Examinations of the Previous Principles.'

In times when crude, injurious, painful methods of therapeutics were prevalent, Master Hahnemann introduced a very fine, gentle, subtle, and dynamic system of medicine. He put forward his new doctrine of 'Similia Similibus Curentur' (Likes cure Like) in contrast with the age-old doctrine of Contraria Contraris Curentur (Dislikes cure Dislikes).

The practical application of this new doctrine demanded a very careful study of the effects of medicines employed in infinitesimal doses on healthy human beings. These medicines if applied on the very basis of the nature's law of cure '*A weaker dynamic affection is permanently extinguished in living beings by a stronger one if the later whilst differing in kind is very similar to the former in its manifestations*' in patients with sufferings similar to the effects of these medicines they could remove the disease symptoms and cure the individuals from the disease.

These effects in the form of symptoms were very minute, subtle, peculiar, uncommon, characteristic and even queer. Hence it became very essential to study these drug diseases (effects of the medicines on healthy provers). It was also important to study carefully effects which the disease agents produced individually on in different persons, so that both could be compared and diseases successfully treated. As time passed numerous medicines were discovered, Dr. Hahnemann and other pioneers like Dr. Constantine Hering, Dr. J. T. Kent proved, verified various remedial agents and thus the Pandora of homeopathy bundled up thousands of medicines with lakhs of symptoms. With so many medicines and such huge number of symptoms, it was very important to understand the dynamic healing concept of homeopathy and study the dynamic activity of medicines on human beings before the application of this system of medicine was undertaken. Many pioneering keen minds put untiring efforts towards the pursuit of this knowledge and very successfully applied the system of therapeutics. The coming generations unfortunately found it to be a system needing tremendous endeavour for its successful application in diseases.

The provings established an 'ideal' a 'perfect' picture of the drug diseases, but in reality it was difficult to perceive this ideal picture, because disease at a particular point of time didn't manifest itself so full and complete. Although different individuals underwent varied sufferings and diseases expressed themselves with multiple manifestations, it was difficult to appreciate these 'personal pictures' of the diseases. Hence by many later generation physicians, their acquired knowledge proved futile when it came to the actual application of the law, and when they had to actually select a remedy, they found themselves in a pond of innumerable difficulties. There were many difficulties on this stage where they had to perform as medical professionals. The pathological prescribing started. Physicians went on to prescribe specific remedies or favourite remedies for specific ailments. And this was the reason, which lead to the death of homeopathy in many parts of the world. Homeopathy lost its individuality, integrity and finally the identity.

These difficulties continued in the later generations too and the present day homeopaths have to come face to face with them. The system being highly refined, needs only a refined way of practicing. It is practically difficult to identify and locate similar effects produced under ideal conditions in healthy individuals in the diseased patients. Not that the manifestations of the disease didn't exist as they did in the Materia Medica (record of homeopathic provings) but they were veiled up due to multiple factors. And we find the present generation of homeopathic graduates go on to prescribe homeopathic combinations or formulas of the so called experienced physicians (who are their *Gurus*) whose experience seems to have heightened only a little even after decades of homeopathic practice. The face of homeopathic prescribing has evolved into a not very beautiful one and there are many other factors, which have been responsible for distorting this face.

We shall now take a look into these factors that are 'bitter realities' or more correctly practical problems in Homeopathic Prescribing:

1.   In most cases the patient lacks self-observation, the patient himself is not able to perceive the finer expressions of the disease. Many times along with this non-observation there is also a mal-observation on his part because of which the physician is mislead and has difficulty in perceiving true picture of the disease.

2.   Even if the manifestations of the disease are 'observed' by

the patient in vast majority of cases but the patient isn't medically trained to 'understand' what he 'observes' and finally he cannot convey it rightly to the physician. On the other hand patients from the educated class may create problems for the physician by making use of wrong medical terminologies very confidently. They describe and theorize their disease on the basis of certain wrong 'medical concepts,' which conceive and evolve in their minds over a period of time, practically making things very difficult for the physician.

3. Illiterate patients and patients from the lower socioeconomic strata are extremely poor in observation and also lack the intelligence to observe peculiar symptoms, which are so significant for making a proper homeopathic prescription.

4. In many cases the patient comes with complaints at a time when the disease has not fully expressed itself because it is not fully evolved. Hence the disease manifestations haven't come out in full. At times these manifestations are chocked with some crude household remedies or the 'over the counter drugs' making things more difficult for the homeopathic physician.

5. The hard fact—It is observed that in reality the diseases often never express in full bloom as the provings of the medicine on a healthy prover.

6. Patient being much distressed is not in a physical and mental state of telling his complaints to the physician.

7. Conveying every minor peculiarity of his sufferings is not really important for a patient and hence he misses out on many things. The patient doesn't realize the importance of many small things because he thinks them 'insignificant' or 'trivial' and hence doesn't feel the least necessity of conveying them to the doctor. Dr. Kent says, "The patients generally

call attention to the commonest things, while it is strange and peculiar things that guide the remedy."

8.   The patients who are entirely new to the science and approaching the physician for the first time, those never being oriented with homeopathy, pose as a great hurdle in the path of prescribing. The influence of approach of modern medicine in 'examining' rather than 'interrogating' makes them feel that the system is strange or weird because of which he may show disinterest and look with contempt at a method of investigating the disease which is so scientific.

9.   Even patients well aware about principles and approach of the science towards dealing with the diseases are at failure to perceive their own sufferings and thus cannot report to the physician.

10. Patients often have their own priorities which they stress upon repeatedly and want the physician to cure first, for they are distressed and hence they miss on other symptoms

11. Materia Medica is so vast and it is not as simple as prescribing an antipyretic for fever or an allopathic hypertensive for high blood pressure as is the case with antipathic mode of treatment. In the science of homeopathy it is always prescribing for the 'diseased person', selecting from the magnum materia medica a remedy that matches with him. One has to study and match so many 'drug pictures' from the materia medica with the 'diseased patient.' One has to select a remedy that perfectly and very closely matches with that of the patient.

12. This selection of the homeopathic remedy has to be based on the difficult and stringent guidelines in the 'Organon of Medicine' if cure is to be achieved, this has always bean an Herculean task.

13. There has to be a qualitative analysis; this is a single long thread that follows homeopathic prescribing. One has to be perfect, complete, upto the mark in everything — observation, perception, analysis, evaluation, knowledge of materia medica and homeopathic philosophy and also in the application of this knowledge.

14. 'For an ideal cure the physician has to make an ideal prescription in most un-ideal conditions.' Be has to be refined in mind, keen, astute, tactful, and quick to be able to be 'Manage a Prescription'.

15. Not always do the close relatives of the patient accompany him. Many times the ones who accompany are often 'negligent fathers' while the mothers are busy in the kitchen at home. Often the person who has been assigned the job of taking the patient to the doctor even doesn't know what the patient is suffering from; in higher classes he is often an indifferent servant, maid or even the driver.

16. Often the 'diseased individual' comes and drops down his head on the table in front of you moaning in pain, and saying feebly "I have fever and this headache what should I do of it? It is paining so much. Doctor do something, relieve me." That is it, that's the diseased individual for the physician and he has to prescribe for it. The patient cannot describe his sufferings for he feels there isn't anything except fever and headache and a homeopathic physician is expected to make an instants yet a correct prescription. Now how to make a scientific homeopathic prescription is a mighty question. If patients are children, they simply cannot express the symptoms and often mislead with all positive 'YES' answers to most of the leading questions (which often become necessary to ask in case of children) and with their negative answers to the questions which they are predetermined to answer in negative for no obvious reasons.

17. Often patients coming from other physicians (ayurvedic, allopathic as well as homeopathic physician) have a complex symptom picture and due to the change in the original symptom picture it becomes difficult to perceive the true symptom picture and make the right prescription. The symptoms of the patient subside due to some drugs prescribed by the previous physician or the over-the-counter drugs consumed by him. Patients usually 'Do something' so that the symptoms change.

18. Patients miss out on alternating symptoms and on the complaints that appear periodically.

19. Some symptoms become so much a part of the patients that they have 'accepted' them as a part and parcel of their living and they don't really feel the need to mention these symptoms, which may be most important for making a prescription.

20. Some patients are shy, reserved, others secretive and due to this many things don't reach the physician. False modesty and shame often conceal many things. Female patients may hesitate to convey gynecological symptoms to the physician and male patients may not express symptoms of the sexual sphere, which are surely significant in making a homeopathic prescription.

21. Sometimes indolence and forgetfulness of the patient act as a major block in prescribing.

22. Exaggeration of complaints on part of the patient with a consideration that the physician will give 'high power' drugs and he will be relieved of their sufferings instantly is one more obstacle. Kent says, "patients exaggerate to induce the physician to depict their suffering in lively colours and make use of exact terms to induce the physician to relieve them promptly."

23. Often the close relatives or people accompanying the patient take extra initiative to express patient's complaints or give account of the history of his sufferings so as to make an impression on the physician. The patient who is in a suffering state and often carries in his mind a not so clear picture of his own sufferings and gives a positive not even without giving a proper ear to what they are saying, thereby fully misguiding the physician.

24. In acute cases exposure to wine, coffee, night watching, mental and physical exertion, an exposure to any external influence masks the case.

These are a few bitter realities, which have never been addressed and need to be addressed on some intellectual platform. We must find solutions to these practical problems. It is perhaps the need of the day.

How to rise above all these practical problems, and how to make a correct prescription given that all the above things will always dominate homeopathic prescribing is what the further chapters of the book attempt to unveil.

∎

CHAPTER 2

THE EXPERT PRESCRIBER

DEFINITION

'You can be an Expert Prescriber' is one who not only possess an indepth knowledge of homeopathy as a science but is also able to skillfully use in making a quick yet a correct scientific homeopathic prescription for every condition within the domain of similia on the available (limited) expressions of the diseased individual, in the existing adverse, unsupportive circumstances and the prevailing prescribing situation he is into and that too without the aid of specialized diagnostic or therapeutic tools and most importantly staying well inside the premises of the homeopathic principles, given the fact that many perils limit him and principles restrict him in many ways.

EXPLANATION

Many a physician can gain mastery over knowledge however vast it may seem but only a few are able to intellectually use it for the benefit of their patients, for achieving a radical cure. This is because although the armamentarium of their knowledge is full with the homeopathic ammunition they don't possess the skill to use this ammunition, which is of utmost importance. Skill is something that can be developed, infact imbibed on the basis of some inherent qualities giving due attention to certain things, making some fixed logical norms and attending some practical problems while treating a case. Again, it is so important that all this is done at pace, for the patient in Suffering Bus is in much of a hurry to give you any time. He is eager to override his sufferings and reach the destination of health fast and quick.

The physician on the responsible driver's seat, has to make his patient reach the destination fast and importantly without any accidents on route. For this, he needs to be a well-trained artist. His road is often narrowed by many limitations, restrictions and holds many hurdles in the form of practical difficulties and unsupportive situations. He can only reach the destination if he applies his skill on the path of principles.

Any short cuts or byways may only lead to accidents. So he needs to train himself well, achieve the skill and mend his knowledge into a more practical and applicable one so that he successfully drives his patient to the ultimate destination of health and cure. That is why he needs to be an expert prescriber, a master Homeopath who is well trained, skillfull, practical, able and competent enough to carry on the above responsibility courageously and efficiently. The aid of diagnostic and therapeutic tools can only make him a mere creeper, a dependent person. A greater dependence on these aids is likely to weaken him and blunt his intelligence. They should only ease his way.

He needs to develop and sharpen his own tool, which, is always ready for his help in trying times and testing situations. He needs to speak in actions and not just words as many of the physicians do boasting of their knowledge and depicting their achieved, unachieved cures. His cures need to introduce him to the rest of the world and give an account of his exceptional skill, his inherent qualities, exceptional abilities and profound knowledge. Some people are born great, some are made great by fortune, some make themselves great by their actions, their hard endeavour and inputs. We   need to follow such great people and I believe strongly if not great we can definitely become better homeopathic prescribers.

An expert prescriber should focus on Dr. Hahnemann's three points necessary for curing:

- The proper investigation of the disease.

- The proper investigation of the effects of medicine.

- The proper employment of medicines.

And for this, a physician must not only be a true practitioner of the healing art and must posses all the below essentials as per Dr. Hahnemann but he should also acquire, posses and develop certain exceptional qualities.

Requisite qualifications of the true practitioner (as mentioned by Dr. Hahnemann in the Organon of Medicine Sec. 3)

- Knowledge of disease

- Knowledge of medicinal powers

- Knowledge of application of drug knowledge to disease knowledge

- Knowledge of choice of the remedy

- Knowledge of the exact mode of preparation

- Knowledge of exact dose required

- Knowledge of proper repetition of dose
- Knowledge of obstacles to cure and their removal
- Knowledge of (Sec.4)

  things that derange health

  things that cause disease

  their removal from persons in health

More over he should have
(As per Sec 6,83,98 of Organon of Medicine)

- No prejudice
- Sound senses
- Especial circumspection
- Tact
- Knowledge of human nature
- Caution in conducting inquiry
- Patience

Besides these qualities an expert prescriber must possess certain exceptional qualities, which can really make him a Master Prescriber.

THE EXCEPTIONAL QUALITIES

SINCERE DESIRE

A strong and sincere desire to become an expert, a master in prescribing is essential to gain an expertise in the art of prescribing. Further a physician must have an eager desire to over come all the difficulties, adversities and practical problems and zeal to do best within limitations and restrictions of the science. In the absence of this strong desire, all the qualities shall be futile.

DETERMINATION

The physician must have the firmness of purpose and a resolution to be a Master prescriber. He should be determined to win over diseases coming his way.

DEVOTION AND DEDICATION

Unless one devotes oneself to the task of acquiring the skill he can never achieve the highest ideal of cure. One has to throw oneself fully into this task and a full dedication to this purpose is extremely important if something substantial is to be really achieved.

GRIT

A prescriber has to undergo many trying situations and testing times which can give him shudders. Only quality courage and endurance can help him to withstand the trials and tribulations of homeopathic practice and make him pass all the acid tests which shall only make him a more stronger and confident physician.

RESILIENCE

Resilience is the quality of quickly recovering to original shape or condition after being pulled, pressed or crushed. This power of recovering quickly is essential because in practice many times things disturb and discourage you. The disappointments pull you down in many ways. This can affect the competence, capabilities and skills of the physician. Hence, one needs to be buoyant, only then can he remain unaffected by the above things.

INQUISITIVENESS

There should be a basic inquisitiveness, which can surely help a physician in investigating a particular case and exploring the science. The spirit to know more of new and unexplored things should be an undying one.

POSITIVE ATTITUDE

Most importantly, a physician should look at things with a positive frame of mind. Take success or failures only in the right spirits. He must walk out of failures with a positive helpful conclusion. A physician must view and approach every new case with a positive mind setup.

COOL TEMPERAMENT

The huge expectations of a rapid and permanent cure, the critical situations, acute emergencies, and too much of a work load can make a physician agitated, nervous and occasionally angry which may effect his competence levels, his work, the selection of the right remedy; hence a homeopathic physician who intends to have a mastery over prescribing needs to have a cool temperament as the greatest quality. He should 'keep himself cool in every situation.'

Besides all these, introspection and retrospection can only give him a chance to improve and become better and better.

CHAPTER 3

THE PHYSICIAN'S PREPARATION

To be a proficient prescriber, the ground level preparations are essentially important. The feeding of the human prescribing computer (Physician's reason-gifted mind) with the vital knowledge of homeopathic materia medica, knowledge of homeopathic philosophy and the constant sharpening of the logical skills are things indispensable to homeopathic prescribing. With more and more experience the knowledge is continuously processed by the mental faculties because of which, intellect is not only sharpened but also enriched with essential 'practical knowledge'. Thus one gets the homeopathic wisdom. And mind evolves into a true 'homeopathic reason-gifted mind.'

The development of a logical thinking is something that should be continually encouraged. This is a self-process and should be consciously chased by the physician. And it can only be done with habit formation, with a conscious realization within oneself to connectedly study things, to correlate the happenings, to understand the cause-effect relationships, to see things in various views. A physician has to develop a holistic homeopathic vision.

F - 3

It can be done by constant questioning, arguing with self, going into the why, what, how of everything. Cardinally the feeding of images constituted in the mental generals, physical generals, characteristic particulars, and uncommon, characteristic peculiar symptoms of the remedies. It is important to understand the 'vital force' the 'essence' of every remedy.

Now the question to many is what exactly is the image of the remedy. To make it simple whatever 'memories of a remedy' whatever 'pictures', or peculiar points that are retained in the mind after repeated reading of the remedy over the period of time is the image of the remedy. It is a simple remembrance. The image is something that doesn't have a specific outline but some vaguely sketched figure. One should study the points on which remedies stand apart, the distinguishing points, the finer discrimination in remedies. You have to 'diagnose' every remedy in your mind and this diagnosis is made on certain points. This needs to be learnt. It is important to study and understand the parallelism in remedies, also the family likeness of groups, the organ affinities and brotherhood of images of remedies of particular group (for example Kali group – Kali-c., Kali-bi., Kali-br.,), the fellow companion images of remedies (example Calc. and Bar-c.).

The only thing that is left over after this is the recording of the case, collecting minutest details and when this collection is about to be completed the 'feed back mechanism' of our trained computer should spring out before us the probable remedies and in many cases even the 'Simillimum' (if mind has been trained as above). One cannot escape the method hence we must go ahead with the analysis and evaluation of symptoms and also construct a totality. After one separates the characteristics of the case, analyzes and evaluates the symptoms, with one single reading into the totality one can be just there at the right remedy. But the 'physician's preparation' as above is very important.

It is important that the language in which the disease expresses itself is learned fully and completely and then only can one become a fluent prescriber. It is also important for the physician to feed the logic of homeopathy, the technique, the method of investigating a patient, principles of prescribing (see further section); all these key threads in his system. Key to making a correct prescription lies in your correct appreciation of the distinctive features of various remedies and your patient. You have to understand the variance, the disparity and the similarity. A homeopath's readiness for hard work, his braving to conquer knowledge, and eagerness to verify the nature's law can yield him great results.

FOLLOWING REFERENCE ARE OF GREAT USE

Materia Medica

- Dictionary of Homeopathic Materia Medica by Clarke.
- Kent's Lectures on Homeopathic Materia Medica.
- Drug Pictures by Tyler.
- A Synoptic Key of Materia Medica by C. M. Boger.
- Allen's Keynotes.

Books in which practical guidelines are given

- Organon of Medicine, sixth edition, Dr. Samuel Hahnemann.
- The Principles and Practice of Homeopathy, Dr. M. L. Dhawale.
- The Principles and Art of Cure by Homeopathy, Dr. Herbert Roberts.
- The Genius of Homeopathy, Stuart Close.
- Lectures on Homeopathic Philosophy, Dr. J. T. Kent.

Only he can evolve into a perfect prescriber who is ready to remain a student of homeopathy all through his life. Perfection is not an end in itself but a continuous process. The secrets of an excellent prescribing are unveiled gradually to every one as one goes deeper and deeper into the science.

■

CHAPTER 4

PRINCIPLES OF PRESCRIBING

If one is really desirous of becoming a good prescriber it is essential that his prescriptions are not only rooted to the strong ground of homeopathic principles but they are also based on principles which we can conveniently call the principles of prescribing. These principles always need to be followed while one makes a homeopathic prescription so that the prescription turns out to be a correct one.

THE VALUABLE PRINCIPLES OF PRESCRIBING

1. Always prescribe for the 'Diseased individual' and not for the disease alone. Prescribe for the 'Individualized disease'. To be more specific prescribe for the individuality of the patient.

2. Always focus on the uncommon, characteristic, peculiar symptoms of the diseased individual. These symptoms that are personal to the patient should always be the basis of the homeopathic prescription.

3. Keep hunting for the queer, rare and strange symptoms. There is nothing more valued than these symptoms in prescribing.

4. The selection of remedy should always be based on the uncommon symptoms. Even one uncommon symptom may form the basis of prescription in acute prescriptions.

5. Multiple common symptoms in a case sometimes go on to make a peculiar symptom picture (Totality) in an individual where no uncommon symptoms are available.

6. In fevers always prescribe for generals of the patient. Prescriptions may at times be based on just the pathological generals.

7. In chronic prescribing the order of importance should be miasm, mental state, thermal modality, mental generals, physical generals and characteristic particulars respectively.

8. Never prescribe on incomplete data. Try to gather as much information as one can through questioning and cross-questioning before making a prescription.

9. Your prescription should always satisfy the knowledge bank inside you, your self- beliefs and homeopathic value system imbibed by you. And if it does so, it is bound to be a correct prescription.

10. Never ever stick, be obsessed or prejudiced with any one school of prescribing—Kentian, Boger, Boenninghausen etc. Never be stubborn on giving importance and advocating a particular philosophy and with that prepossession don't just prescribe for mentals, or merely physical generals, characteristic particulars or pathological generals. Give consideration and due importance to symptoms in all the spheres and prescribe for the 'Picture', the 'Portrait', the 'Totality of symptoms' in which all the above symptoms have their due share.

11. A physician in order to master homeopathic prescribing must hold equal regard for every philosophy, every school of prescribing. No physician who says "I prescribe simply on mentals, or pathological generals and I have a mastery over it," can ever be called a Master homeopathic prescriber.

12. In cases especially acute deviations from the state of health give utmost importance to the 'Cause' followed by 'Modalities', 'Sensations,' 'Concomitants' respectively and lastly the 'Location.'

13. The doctrine of not prescribing for the chronic and acute trouble together should always be remembered. Kent says, "Never prescribe for any two conditions unless they be complicated."

14. Never prescribe for a symptom, or simply the disease prescribe for the patient, treat the patient not the disease and your prescription wi!! automatically be a correct one.

SUGGESTIONS FOR PRESCRIBING

1. In chronic cases after the case is recorded however sure you may be of the Simillimum never be too ambitious to prescribe a remedy instantaneously. Curb you eagerness, your 'psoric itch' to do so. Always aim to study the case in totality. First analyze, evaluate and study the case, prepare a Totality, construct the patient's image on paper fully. Refer different Materia Medicas for comparison and drug differentiation compare the 'image' of your patient with the 'images of the remedies' you hold in your mind through your study and knowledge and then find out the most 'Simillimum.'

THE PRACTICAL SUGGESTIONS

- Always aim at studying the case in totality.

- Don't be too ambitious.

- Never be in a hurry to prescribe.

- When in doubt wait.

- Always go for the common first.

- In chronic cases, 'Miasms' are the final decider.

- In acute cases, the Thermals and Generals are the final decider.

- A placebo for a complex, incomplete and non-recognizable picture.

2.   'When in doubt wait'—this frequently used axiom in homeopathy is usually applied to the second prescription, but I feel it is applicable to the first prescription also. I advise when a physician is in doubt over the selection of one remedy or if the patient's picture doesn't fit into any of the probable remedies, and if some remedies only partially resemble the patient one must wait for some time. Some symptoms of the patient, which may be the key symptoms for the prescription may have yet to make an appearance in the patient because the disease in the patient when he approaches you is not fully evolved. So wait for some time and some new important symptoms may come to the surface and you can make satisfactory prescription. Wait for the true image of the disease evolve.

3.   Never be in a hurry to ride the bus of patient's suffering. Except course in acute cases like high fever, food poisonings etc. you must assess the condition of the patient and verify if

actually you have the time to wait. Otherwise one has to prescribe on the available data if the situation demands an emergency prescription.

4. A placebo should be administered when symptom picture is complex, complicated, incomplete, indiscrete, scattered and non-recognizable.

5. A remedy is never contraindicated in homeopathy but it is always indicated in homeopathy. When making a choice of remedy think on positive lines think why a particular remedy is indicated in a case and not why it is not indicated . For example—A remedy like Gelsemium should not be discarded when all other features match only because the patient is thirsty and the remedy has absence of thirst as the marked feature. Match patient to the remedy and not remedy to the patient. Not all the features of the remedy can be present in the patient but remedy may still be indicated and cure the patient. Selection of remedy should always be a positive conclusion and not a negative derivation. It's the essence of the remedy that should be present in the patient and not all prominent features. This should be clearly remembered and cleverly practiced.

6. When often two or three remedies run close the thermal reaction of the patient becomes the 'decider.' Do give it the utmost significance when you are blocked with two remedies going close to the patient especially in acute cases. In chronic cases the fundamental / dominating Miasm in the patient should be awarded the prime importance.

7. Always 'go for the common first ' think of common remedies first, again think of the common diagnosis first and you are most likely to react the right place the correct remedy and the correct diagnosis. It makes your task simple, clear and easy.

To conclude in a few words –'A balanced all round approach in every way to making a prescription is the key to prescribing'.

■

CHAPTER 5

THE ART OF ACUTE PRESCRIBING

Given the conditions under which one has to make an acute prescription one needs to do it very intelligently. Skillful use of our knowledge can make us a good acute prescriber. This chapter attempts to train a physician in this art. The points described should be carefully noted and adopted.

HISTORY OF THE ACUTE AILMENTS

Skillful extraction of a detailed history from the patient, gathering the 'minutiae' in acute ailments is a much bigger, difficult and a testing task for the physician than the actual selection of the simillimum. A right approach to the 'extraction of the totality' is essential without which, useful information cannot be drilled out.

So a physician should proceed for the inquiry systematically under some fixed heads, keeping in mind the expression of the disease phenomenon (symptoms) in materia medica. Only then can he derive data that shall help him to select a remedy as per the materia medica. The physician must go ahead with the inquiry under the following heads. The relevance and practical utility of 'acute history' towards the selection of the right remedy has been elaborated further in the chapter.

The acute history should be collected under the following heads

- The Probable cause
- Onset of the complaints
- Progression
- Exact sensations
- Modalities
- Concomitants
- Exact location

THE PROBABLE CAUSE

No homeopathic mind is left untouched with the untold utilities of the cause in making a correct homeopathic prescription. The immense usefulness of the 'cause' lies in the fact that when many a times no uncommon peculiar sensations, no modalities, neither the concomitants are available in an acute case and when a totality cannot be constructed, the cause and the common symptoms of the patient unite and bring forth a 'remedy image'.

A prescription simply based on the cause, in many cases proves to be a wonderful one. Irrespective of the sufferings of the patient, a remedy based on the cause can offer a sure shot cure and even relieve those symptoms that you may not found under the remedy in the materia medica.

For example a known cause like shouting by parents giving rise to particular suffering can be relieved by remedies like Cina, Ignatia. In a case of fall and mechanical injury a remedy like Arnica can relieve any suffering that results from the injury. Dr. Hahnemann and other pioneers of homeopathy have stressed hard on the treatment of the cause in acute ailments.

Other Examples

A typical case of watery summer diarrhoea, associated with body pains and mild nausea, so many remedies come into fray. With the absence of any uncommon characteristic, peculiar symptom it becomes difficult for a homeopathic healer to select a remedy. Here the assessment of cause is very important and it is really important to find out whether there has been a history of eating in eateries, hotels, unclean places, marriage, functions etc.

If there is any such history, which is suggestive of ptomaine poisoning (food poisoning) a remedy like Ars-alb. proves to be the correct prescription. And if there is no such history and only a history of an exposure to sun, or of consuming cold drinks in hot environment, and where it seems to be an apparent case of sun stroke a remedy like Bry. should be the right remedy. Here with all the common symptoms but established cause and the right diagnosis, a scientific homeopathic prescription could be made.

So, where only common symptoms are present and no modalities and concomitants can be found in a case, a cause like the 'recent exposure' should always come to the respite of the physician. If the patient does not communicate, recollect or directly point out at the cause, it is the physician who should recollect whether there has been a sudden change in the weather or temperature a day or two before. He should recall in mind whether there was a rainy or cloudy weather or scorching heat or a biting cold or a storm a day or two before which may be the cause for the patient's complaints and also a good guide to the remedy. Here the physician has to consider the 'probabilities and possibilities' and even if the patient doesn't give a direct history or reference of any such exposure a physician has to explore them and consider them seriously.

So '*Prescribe for the weather if you cannot prescribe for the patient or his disease'* is a modern day mantra which a homeopathic physician should remember. A physician should always keep in his mind a list of 'seasonal remedies', i.e. remedies which are usually indicated in a particular season weather and it will be very practical to select one from amongst them, the one that is suitable to your patient. In the absence of reliable information a physician has to intellectually ascertain the probable cause himself and simply prescribe for it.

A Million Dollar Question

What to do when a cause is not traceable and the patient presents himself with all the common symptoms?

Here physician's being update, his circumspection offers a dear help. He needs to be aware about the existing diseases prevalent in the area. He should update himself through the newspapers, pamphlets and announcements by the local municipal corporations or other governing bodies. He should be read afresh regarding the diseases and see if he finds any symptoms of the disease in the patient, he should try to establish the diagnosis and interrogate the cause, which will be immensely helpful for a prescription. The common symptoms of the disease also furnish a picture and point to a homeopathic remedy this is one rare fact but needs to be given attention in prescribing. Simultaneously a physician's search for a 'genus epidemicus' should be on and he should be ready with it. He can choose a genus epidemicus on the basis of the symptoms of a particular disease prevalent in his area at a particular point of time.

MODE OF ONSET

Its important to study the mode of onset of the complaints because the manner in which the complaints set in or make their appearance, the manner in which they develop and evolve characterize the case and can prove significant in selection of remedy. For example in a general complaint like headache suppose one is not able to trace back the cause is the modalities or the concomitants, then with just the location and sensation with us we may select a remedy like Bell, where there is a sudden and violent onset of complaints and in a slow gradual developing case of headache, Gels. may be indicated.

PROGRESSION

The progression of the complaints is very important in deciding a prescription. In the presence of all the common symptoms interrogation about the disease process should suggest you a remedy. For example: the colds in Merc-sol. are of ascending type and have a tendency to settle in eyes, they travel upwards while the colds of Ars. travel from nose downwards to the posterior nares and are thus are descending type of colds. Like wise complaints in Sepia ascend. Complaints proceed from above downwards in Kalm., and in Led. they ascend, in Rhus-t. they move from left to right. In Puls. and Kali-bi. the pains shift. Thus All these moves and shifts point towards the prescription.

SENSATIONS

The 'sensations' too are important in homeopathy. No physician can ever underestimate the value of sensations, which need to be precisely taken a note and perceived in exactness so that the individuality of the patient's suffering is brought out. In homeopathic materia medica a variety of sensations characterizing various remedies can be observed like burning pains of Ars., Apis, Phos., splinter like sensation of Hep., and Nit-ac. Tearing pains of Rhus-t. Stitching pains of Bry., Choking sensation of Cact.

A physician should make the patient describe, the exact sensation. He should tell him to express the sensation in his own language. Here a physician should be well versed with the local dialect and local terminologies for sufferings. Empathy always helps a physician to feel the patient's sensation. By putting himself in the patient's shoes and with a little insight he should judge what exactly is the patient going through and collect the peculiarities.

MODALITIES

Well who doesn't know what the modalities directly offer a homeopathic prescription, undoubtedly the right remedy. Yes they make it a perfect one. In the order of importance, the modalities stand next to the cause. They beautify the sensations to present before us an elegant totality. When nothing seems to point to a particular remedy modalities often guides the correct road to following remedy. These modalities should mainly be investigated under the heads—Time modalities, Positional modalities, Thermal modalities, Seasonal modalities, Discharge modalities-sweat, sleep, stools, Other modalities - draft, touch, odour, foods, sound, light which may be the aggravating factors and need to be considered. If you are not able to find out modalities one can 'demonstrate modalities' for example the patient with pain in legs may be told to walk, to get up, to sit up thus on the spot inquiry can be made. You may put off or switch on the fan in your chamber and know the patient's experience whether he feels better or worse. Such and other practical methods may be thought upon by the physician to find out modalities of the patient.

CONCOMITANTS

Concomitants are the symptoms, which are present along with the chief complaints although they have no direct relationship with the chief complaints except for their time of appearance. Concomitants help to draw the picture of the patient. Concomitants may be general concomitants like thirst, appetite, sweat, sleep, some general sensations like heaviness, weakness, or burning. Again in the patient there may be 'evident mental concomitants' like irritability, weepy, depression etc. They also include the thermals of the patient, his desire and aversion for covers and simultaneous sufferings relating to other parts. Boenninghausen has given a lot of importance to the concomitants.

Tongue the remedy pointer

I know this special sense organ of the human body by another name and that is a 'Remedy.' Pointer because in many of my cases it has helped me to select the proper remedy and discard other few other that were running close. Tongues of various remedies help a physician in the final choice. In Materia Medica we have very characteristic tongues like dry white coated tongue of Bry., a thick white coated tongue of Ant-c., a mapped tongue with a triangular red tip of Rhus-t. With limited symptoms, tongue aids in prescribing a particular remedy.

EXACT LOCATION

C.M. Boger has given the importance to the exact location and it is also an essential part of the acute totality. Its important to know exact location of the affection. Often we may see in a particular case of acute exacerbation of arthritis that the left hip and right shoulder are paining which strongly point to a remedy like Led.

If the tonsils are affected Hep. and Merc. emerge as two prime remedies and the prescriptions can be made just by inquiring about the thermals. In a case of acute abdomen pain more localized to epigastric region point to Nux-v. and pain all over abdomen to China if other symptoms agree. So knowing the 'exact location' and not just the part affected is important.

MAKING THE DIAGNOSIS

I wish to place a paradox here 'Diagnosis besides its known significance and utilities in homeopathy also helps to select a remedy.'

I substantiate the above statement with a few examples.

If a particular pain is diagnosed as a congestive pain one can think of remedies like Bell. and Bry. while if it is a neuralgic pain which is ameliorated by pressure, bending double and warmth one may thing of remedies like Mag-p., Coloc. etc.

Diagnosis in many cases can even directly aid in selection of a simillimum. In a case of bilateral swelling on face with fever and profuse salivation if you know your surgery well you can surely diagnose that it is a case of acute parotitis.

And even with limited symptomatology a remedy like Merc. can be selected as the location of the disease that is established thoroughly along with the profuse salivation point out to it . Thus understanding the disease phenomenon can aid in the prescription. But the symptoms of the patient are always our infallible guide.

EXAMINATION OF THE PATIENT

'A patient well examined is half cured.' I have designed this modern day adage because the complete examination of the patient can really make the job of prescribing easy for the physician and cure his patient quick and fast. By examination, a physician may encounter certain features of the diseased individual. And many things for making a correct prescription may be revealed to him through examination. The examination of the patient should not only be complete i. e. from head to foot but it should also be based on Materia Medica. The physician should also examine the patient from the point of view of Materia Medica and try to search for the characteristic features of the remedy in the patient. One should look for the 'usual features of the remedies.'

THE INQUIRY

The physician should make an inquiry in a case with respect to Materia Medica. Kent says "one of the most important things in securing the image of a sickness is to preserve in simplicity what the patient tells us in his own way unless he digresses from important things and talks about things that are foolish and not to the point."

Silence speaks a lot. When the patient is not referring to certain point, suggest the physician that he should deeply inquire into them. On inquiry if negative symptoms are found they are important, for example; painless diarrhoea. Remember, the 'Nothing in a patient points to something.'

PATIENT EDUCATION

A physician must educate his patients that the simplest and minutest details about his ailments are always important for him. A physician should to be able to take him into full confidence and communicate to him in an effective manner about the homeopathic approach to a case. Only that will prompt the patient to recollect and tell every small thing about his sickness. Most physicians give less importance to this sort of education and awareness.

It is infact the duty of the physician is to not only tell the above things but also firmly impress upon the patient's mind the following things

1. The symptoms that he expresses shall be the only basis of the medicine/treatment given to him.

2. They shall alone make him free from his illness quickly and fully.

3. They are very important and a remedy can only be perfectly selected if the information by the patient is right .

THE PRESCRIBING SYMPTOM

It is the symptom on which the physician has to base a remedy. Often physician has to choose a remedy resembling the 'The single symptom totality.' It is one symptom in a case, which solicits our attention by carrying itself proudly in a case when the other symptoms are complex and confusing.

Example 'Great thirst for chilled drinks but are vomited out as soon as they reach stomach' should call for Ars. as the remedy.

DRAWING THE ACUTE PICTURE CONSTRUCTING THE TOTALITY

The acute totality of the patient should be constructed under the following heads in the following manner and order. Only then can a characteristic picture of the patient emerge on the paper.

1. GENERALS

These are the generals of the patient, which are present in the chronic as well as acute stages. They remain unchanged in the acute stage. Here following should be included:

Mentals

Thirst

Sweats

Appetite

Sleep

General sensations

2. SECTOR TOTALITY

Cause: Causative factor, Exciting, Precipitating cause

Modalities: Aggravation & Amelioration.

Sensation

> Concomitants: General Concomitants.
>
> Mental & Physical.
>
> Particular Concomitants.

Location

DIFFICULTIES ENCOUNTERED

I wish to give this paper a touch of reality with this example:

A child comes to you with high fever, bodyache and headache. There is no appreciable cause in the case, no history of any exposure, neither any modalities of his pains. You ask him about his appetite, he has come to you at 11 a.m. and is yet to have his food and can't really tell you whether he will have a desire for it when he goes home. You ask him about thirst and he vaguely tells you he had one or two glasses of water since morning from this information you can deduce nothing about his thirst. You ask him about stools and he tells you due to fever he didn't get the sensation. You ask about covers he tells I feel like taking them but after a while I feel I should remove them.

There are no other features in the case and the physician is still expected to prescribe. This happens very frequently. This is the real test of the physician, how to prescribe is a million dollar question? What to do now a Physician asks himself?

This section is about how to deal all such situations. Many times the patients do come with an aura of the disease condition and with very little symptoms, because the disease hasn't developed yet.

The reality is, many times **none** of the above is available – neither the causation, the characteristic modalities nor the sensations, the concomitants which are essential for making a prescription, they are no where to be seen in the patient .

THE SOLUTION

The physician has to keep in mind that, a suffering patient, visits to you with most of the essential constituents of the totality. Like our medicines, the inimical force also proves itself on human beings by producing individual symptoms. Never get discouraged if you get nothing. Don't get disappointed, make a final try. You are bound to get 'something', the uncommon, characteristic peculiarities are always there. But, either the patient has not observed them or he is unable to perceive them or communicate it to the physician. When these things are not available to a physician he has to simply make them available for himself. And this is very much possible. He doesn't have to depend on the patient for this. One has to simply 'dig the totality.' If the physician is not able to construct the totality on the available data, he has to 'dig the totality' and for this he needs to develop his personal skill.

Examination plays the key

The physician should first of all examine the patient from head to foot. He must examine every system not only from the diagnostic point of view but also with the aim of discovering some peculiar signs in the patient, some physical evidences, which may well be used to prescribe a remedy. After examining the patient he may find out many peculiar things in the patient like dry hot skin, facial peculiarities like the flushed or pale face, a red tipped, mapped, ragged tongue, a dry cracked peeling off lips, sordes, fever blisters, aphthae at the edges of tongue, congested tonsils, fiery red throat, swollen elongated uvula, the intermittent rapid pulse, or bradycardia , a raised the blood pressure, the sweats, congestion or pallor in eyes, swollen nose, wheezes in chest , rapidly beating heart, hot palms, sweaty soles, rumbles in abdomen, tenderness in abdomen, enlargement of liver, enlargement of glands, generalized lymphadenopathy. All these may give one some physical signs so as to make a totality.

Important Tips

Often it is the patient or his relative who takes you to the remedy, so give a decent ear to what a patient and his relatives say. They will take you to the seat of the sufferings prompting you to select a remedy accordingly when nothing else is available for prescribing. A patient may say 'mera main problem gale me hai, bas ye thik ho jaye to baki to mamuli hai'. Another me say 'Bas ye sardard hi pareshan kar raha hai bukhar ka to kuch nahi, ye hatodo ki mar band kar dijiye.' He will draw his own portrait before you and tell you what is marked in him and what should serve the basis of your prescription. What is of importance to the patient should also be important for the physician in selecting a remedy. It should serve the basis of 'the selected' remedy. Causal sentences from the patient may give the clue 'I am sweating so much but the fever doesn't seem to come down' that means, 'profuse sweats which don't relieve and one can think of Merc. or Hep. as probable remedies.'

Chronic peculiarities

When practically nothing is available on which a prescription can be based, the prescription can be based on some known Chronic peculiarities like profuse sweats, desires, aversions, chronic thirst because these also belong to the patient as a person and along with some common symptoms characterize the patient.

Complaints of the past

The physician should see if the patient had similar complaints in the past and examine the remedy prescribed at that time which may well offer the cure to the patient this time too. The affection of the patient may be similar like the previous one. Examining the symptoms of the past and enquiry on the basis of those symptoms may also be helpful.

Simultaneous complaints

These should be noted and remedies which cover these complaints may be prescribed. Complaints like dysmenorrhoea, aphthae in mouth, ear pain etc. may be included in the acute totality although they are not related, but occur simultaneously in the patient hence they form the essential part of the patients sufferings.

Synthetic prescriptions

They are very helpful when we find that the patient doesn't fit in any of the remedies and presents a mixed picture of his ailment. Here remedies like Ant., Ars., Mag-s. etc. often come to the physician's rescue. The remedy in totality covers the patient and includes the symptoms not only covered by the individual remedy but also the constituents.

Example

A case of Fever with chills, a thin acrid coryza, with dry cough burning in palates and throat with severe pain in joints aggravated by rest accompanied with excessive weakness. Here two remedies are indicated Rhus-t. and Ars. but the remedy that fits completely into picture is China, Arsenicum which is the perfectly indicated remedy in the case. This aspect of synthetic homeopathy needs to be attended and explored by every homeopathic physician given the limitations in which one has to practice the science. Also give due importance to the **contradictory or the alternating** symptoms which may well guide you to a remedy when there is paucity of symptoms. Experience leads to better understanding of all acute remedies.

TACKLING AGGRAVATION FEARS

More than anything what haunts a homeopathic physician is the fear of aggravation. Even the simillimum may cause the aggravation if the physician commits some folly in selecting the potency and repeating the doses. Often too frequent repetitions and the unsuitable potency cause an aggravation, which is very difficult to over come.

I recommend the following guidelines to the physician so as to prevent the aggravations:

1. Special precaution should be taken in cases of long lasting cough and often a single dose of thirty potency is sufficient to cure the cough. Hahnemann has mentioned that a single dose of thirty potency is sufficient to cure influenza epidemic and a second dose may prove harmful. It is applicable to most cases of cough. If need is felt for repetition because of other associated complaints like fever. Repetition in two hundred potency is less likely to cause an aggravation.

2. In cases of asthma low to medium potencies may be used and repetition should be avoided.

3. Although selection of potency and repetition depends on the susceptibility of the patient and intensity of the complaints, it is observed that cases of skin wonderfully respond to a single dose of thirty potency.

4. In hypersensitive patients one needs to judge the sensitivity by prescribing a placebo. Hypersensitive patients often show a violent reaction to even placebo although the exact reason for this cannot be ascertained.

5. A single dose of constitutional potency or two doses on two consecutive nights at bed time often give a wonderful response in chronic cases without an aggravation.

6. In pathological conditions low potency should be used. If need is felt frequent or infrequent repetition may be done. Often pathological conditions require repetition.

7   Never prescribe the constitutional remedy in acute phase of the disease or acute exacerbation, it may prove deadly.

Here it is noteworthy that a slight aggravation is always a welcome sign for a homeopathic physician and should not be feared. Here the patient feels better inspite of the aggravation and he is not in a distressed state. Hence a physician should judge the nature of aggravation and then act accordingly.

REMEDY RESPONSE IN ACUTE AILMENTS

The first greatest indicator that the remedy has acted is 'THE GENERALS IMPROVE'.

The mental disposition of the patient improve.

No new symptoms appear, the old symptoms disappear or may have slight aggravation.

The second great indicator is that the 'PATIENT REPORTS A SLIGHT AGGRAVATION YET IT IS NOT DISTRESSING AND PATIENT FEELS WELL'.

ACCIDENTAL DISCOVERIES

Due importance should be given to the contradictory or the alternating symptoms which may well guide you to a remedy when there is paucity of symptoms.

According to Dr. Roberts more serious the conditions more clear cut are the indications of the remedy. He says, "If we allow ourselves to be guided by these symptoms, we shall probably save the patient, even though the remedy selected on the basis of the symptoms totality may never have been used under like diagnostic conditions before".

Key to prescribing is 'prescribe for your gut feeling' which is generated from your knowledge, experience and intellectual correlation of both. We should see to its work and put efforts so that every time we get the right feeling.

CHAPTER 6

TREATING FEVERS WITH HOMEOPATHY

TREATING FEVER — A CHALLENGE

The successful treatment of fevers by homeopathy is quite difficult even by the experienced physicians. It still remains a challenge posed to the homeopathic fraternity. Only an expert can meet the challenges. The treatment of fevers with homeopathy still remains a riddle to the budding homeopaths and in spite of successfully completing the prescribed curriculum, they are never confident of treating the cases of fever.

It is so unfortunate that practitioners of such a highly logical and effective therapy that is known to have a scientific lookout towards everything find treatment of fevers troublesome, which are of commonest occurrence in the day-to-day practice. A right approach in investigating the patient and selection of the remedy can do wonders. If one is able to treat fevers successfully, a physician can gain full trust of the patient. We have still people carrying doubts whether homeopathy will be able to cure fevers like Typhoid, Malaria.

Master Hahnemann has mentioned a rapid, gentle and permanent restoration of health may it be an acute case like fever or any other chronic ailment. But the reality speaks to the contrary.

Time and again we hear that experience is the best teacher but experience only remains a personal tutor of the person who gets it. Dr. Kent says 'Unless man has truth in his mind his experiences are false, truth in the mind is first and then experiences are good.' If his mind is in a state of truth, experiences are true. You cannot trust the experience of men who do not know what is true neither can they be led into truth by these fallacious experiences. The vast experiences encountered in the practice and the conclusions deduced from these experiences by the people in this science unfortunately keep themselves limited to these experienced people, these veterans in homeopathy.

Infact they should serve as a guiding lamp to others especially to the students. This special section on treatment of fevers is an attempt to highlight the useful guidelines given by master Hahnemann towards treatment of fevers.

THE INQUIRY —IN A CASE OF FEVER

In cases of fever as with other cases, inquiry holds the key. This should be done carefully and deeply. Questioning and cross - questioning should be done so that the correct information is obtained. The basic inquiry remains the same as is the case with other acute ailments. But certain things should be carefully inquired and attended, which are as follows:

Duration

Duration of the fever, i.e. since when is the patient suffering from fever.

Cause

Inquiry should be made about the probable cause, like history of any exposure to sun or cold weather etc.

Type

Continuous, remittent or intermittent- What kind of fever it is? Chills or without chills. Also, a detailed inquiry should be made about all the three stages – chill, heat and sweat.

What is most distressing symptom of the patient should also be inquired into?

One should inspect and examine a patient for the suppurative focus or any other significant finding.

Generals should be carefully gathered like thirst, appetite, sleep, sweat, mentals and other concomitants. General sensation like burning, hot feeling etc. should be inquired. Tongue should be carefully observed.

Look for the 'uncommon in common'.

The symptoms (especially the generals) during afebrile stage are very important in fever they should be taken a note of.

PHYSICAL EXAMINATION

Temperature

Pulse

Blood pressure

Respiratory rate

Chest examination

Abdominal examination- for tenderness, liver, spleen enlargement etc.

Examination of eyes for pallor, icterus, congestion etc.

Examination of ear, nose mouth and tongue, throat.

Inspection: general look of the face and skin like dusky, flushed, pale, swollen, eruptions, dryness etc.

Tenderness of sinuses, frontal, ethmoidal, maxillary.

Lymphatic enlargement.

Systemic examination respiratory system, cardiovascular system, nervous system.

To sum up in Dr. H C Allen's words:

'The symptoms occurring before and during the chill, heat, sweat and apyrexia; the time of occurrence of paroxysm: the parts of the body in which chill first makes its appearance the regularity of its stages the degree or absence of thirst the time of its appearance: as well as the constitutional ailments aroused by the fever are all to be carefully noted'.

HOW TO PRESCRIBE?—Six keys to a successful prescription

1. Prescribe on the 'totality of symptoms' for the, ' conceptual image of the patient' for the, 'personal picture of the patient'.

2. Don't prescribe for the fever alone, don't just make a diagnostic prescription like Arn. or Bapt. for Typhoid, China for Malaria.

3. Prescribe for the 'febrile individual.' Rather than individual fever.

4. Prescribe for generals and you are bound to get favourable results.

5. Prescribe for the seat of the disease, your remedy should be directed towards eradicating the infective focus (inimical force), the cause of fever.

6. Give importance to the system involved and affections of the organs that have lead to fever try to select a remedy having marked action on that particular system if no characteristics are present.

WHEN TO ADMINISTER THE REMEDY IN INTERMITTENT FEVER?

As per Sec. 236 of Organon, 'In these cases the medicine is generally most efficacious when it is administered a short time after the termination of the paroxysm, when the patient has partially recovered from it.'

HOW TO JUDGE THE RESPONSE IN FEVER AND PRESCRIBE ACCORDINGLY?

More than the selection of the remedy it is all the more important to carefully judge the response one gets to the administered remedy. A physician needs to give sufficient time to one remedy before shifting to another even when he doesn't receive a single positive response. He needs to stick to a remedy and for this he should have sufficient courage. He should give chance and time to the remedy. There may be an initial lack of response, (aggravation in fever is less likely) this is because after the remedy is prescribed the natural and artificial disease both are at its peak for some period, hence a 'status quo' can be observed in the patients condition.

The first greatest indicator that the remedy has acted is 'THE GENERALS IMPROVE.'

The second great indicator is that the 'PATIENT REPORTS A SLIGHT AGGRAVATION YET IT IS NOT DISTRESSING AND PATIENT FEELS WELL.' The overall look of the patient will improve he will look less distressed less suffering and more at ease. The mentals and disposition improve.

No new symptoms appear.

The old symptoms disappear or are reduced in intensity.

Patience yields very good results in such cases. Doses administered every three or four hours are expected to give a delayed response with sudden flushing and sweating and fever comes down rapidly. Fevers usually have a 'one night stand' irrespective of their variety and often need 14 to 24 hours for cure, except the Malarial and Typhoid fever. In Malarial fevers it may take two four hours or eight days to break the paroxysm but the range of temperature comes down early.

OTHER RESPONSES

It may happen that fever subsides but the headache or bodyache may persists in such cases a placebo should be continued and if in two to three days the complaints are not ameliorated another remedy may be selected for that particular sector of the symptoms. In cases where fever and other complaints are relieved but cough is aggravated sac-lac or next indicated remedy should be the prescription. If a fever returns after amelioration, it doesn't mean that the remedy is just palliative and needs be changed. Here the generals of the patient are to be observed and if one finds that they are improving and other sufferings like headache and body pains etc. are being ameliorated, one should go for further repetitions. Many times when the disease agent is stronger more repetitions are needed and sometimes in a higher potency.

Many times it does happen that the temperature of the patient is unchanged yet the patient feels better which should be considered a positive response of the remedy. When you realize that the fever is brought to the minimum lowest, like 98.8° F or 99° F (normal being 98.4° F) at such time do not repeat the doses. Repetition may cause an aggravation here. In such case is deranged vital force, is sufficiently restored to a near normal state of harmonious functioning and can over come the rest of the symptoms on its own. Again this 'low range fever' is often the artificial disease, which needs no medicine.

IDEAL RESPONSE

The ideal response in a fever is 'fever coming down slowly by half to one degree over a period of few hours and generals of the patient improving at a faster pace. This should be assessed as an excellent response. In fever frequent repetitions cause a delayed yet sharp quick effect. Ideally a perceptible and continued progress contra-indicates repetition.' The exactly similar remedy once found should not be changed until the change of symptoms forms a new picture of the disease to be again met by its Simillimum.

Dr. Allen says, 'We must prescribe from our Materia Medica as it is. Where we can do no better, we must prescribe on a few symptoms, or an interference or an analogy rather than refuse to prescribe at all. Apply less importance to the local symptoms of the drug and the general symptoms (not generals).' Dr. Hahnemann says in treatment of sporadic or epidemic intermittent fever the whole febrile paroxysms it to be taken into account as a unity, he says that the remedy should correspond to similarity of symptoms of strongest marks and most peculiar alternating state.

But he further mentions that the most appropriate remedy would be that which is homeopathic to the symptoms of the patient's health during the interval between successive paroxysmal attacks of patients disease.

AUXILIARY MEASURES

When one treats fever without direct physiological anti-pyretics used in antipathic mode of treatment, a close monitoring becomes essential and two hourly recording of fever is advised.

F - 5

Special care should be taken in case of paediatric patients. As a general rule patient should be removed to a cool environment. He should take his food and plenty of water and electrolytes. Cold sponging should be done for temperatures above 101° F in children and 102 ° F in adults. For every fever above 101° F cold packs should be applied to the head.

CASES

CASE 1

A case of fever with chills in a child aged 6 years, the temperature fluctuating between 103-104° F, the case was referred from a paediatrician. The patient had undergone allopathic treatment of chloroquine, and antipyretics for last one week without any response. The symptoms were headache, thirstlessness although lips and tongue were dry. The child complained of bitter taste in mouth all the year round. With Puls. 200 three doses every two hours the fever totally subsided in about eight hours. No further repetition was done.

CASE 2

A case of fever with chills, temperature 102° F, TLC19,000 physical findings revealed lymphadenopathy of neck and throat congestion ++. The patient had desire for covers +++, Hep-s. 200 was selected on the basis of this data and repeated 4 hourly, the fever subsided in 36 hours and TLC came down to 7,800 after four days.

CASE 3

A case of Chicken pox with itching and burning, exanthematous eruptions on face, back, chest and extremities almost matured with pus and fluid, came to me. The fever was

99.6° F, pulse was rapid there were small red aphthae on tongue, lips and cheeks, tonsils were enlarged, uvula swollen, profuse salivation on mouth. Thirst moderate, appetite diminished, pain in abdomen were the other symptoms. There was cervical lymphadenopathy. On the basis of the picture Merc-s. in 200 potency four doses in three hours duration were administered. The next day in the morning the patient reported with fair GC, was afebrile, burning and itching reduced, eruptions disappearing, he was given sac-lac for two days and was completely relieved in next two days. This case showed any remedy can cure any disease only if it is prescribed on totality of symptoms.

CASE 4

A married man around 35 years of age came to me in mid summer with fever associated with chills. Temperature recorded was 102° F. Physical examination revealed congestion of throat. He complained of bodyache and no peculiarities were present in the case. To select a remedy was a difficult task. The history revealed that he had joined swimming few days back he was exposed to heat on the way since his timing wers 4-5 p.m. and he immediately took shower to cool down and no sooner he reached the pool. Rhus-t. 200 potency was prescribed three hourly on the basis of the characteristic cause of getting wet chilled when hot. The fever subsided and the patient was well in a day.

CASE 5

A patient came to me with history of fever 100° F ameliorated since he had taken paracetamol tablet a few hours back, his temperature at the clinic was subnormal. He complained of tenesmus off and on with loose watery stools. Tenesmus was only temporarily ameliorated by stools. Simultaneously he had aphthae in mouth and also complained of earache. There were no chills, weakness was ++. With no hesitation I prescribed Merc-s. 200 to him which offered the relief promptly.

CASE 6

A 29 year old house wife came with history of fever with chills since last three days. Peripheral smear for malarial parasite was advised, which was positive for P. vivax. The fever intermitted on alternate days. She had terrible headache and bodyache during the chill stage. Usually in evenings the fever had its onset with chills. The accompanying complaint was yellowish cough since last few days. Thirstlessness was a notable feature in the patient.

Puls. 200 was selected on the basis of the above symptoms by which slowly the paroxysms of the fever were broken and by the end of the week the fever totally subsided after 12 days peripheral smear for malarial parasite was done which was negative.

In none of the given variety of cases so-called 'effectice remedies for fever' were used but simple remedies, which were obviously indicated on the basis of totality were administered which yielded wonderful results in these seemingly difficult cases of fever.

∎

CHAPTER 7

HOW TO INVESTIGATE PATIENT'S MIND ?

First and foremost objective of a physician while investigating the patient's mind, should be to know the mental state of the person because it is this state that represents the *core of the image formed by the physical generals*. The conceptual image of a person cannot be properly sketched unless we have this mental state with us. The primary objective of investigating one's mind is to know him as a person and to portary his 'mental picture'. It is important for us to know the inner man from homeopathic point of view.

THE PRESENT CONCEPTS

The present concepts, which the students and physicians harbour about investigating the mentals is forceful interrogation of patient's mentals through bombarding them with leading questions. Do you get angry? Are you emotional? Do you like company? Do you feel the fear? The answer to all the questions most of the times is a 'yes'. Well who doesn't get angry and doesn't fear anything. It is not the right method by which one goes about investigating the patient's mind.

*I would like to briefly enumerate the present miscon-
ceptions which vast majority of physicians carry about
investigating the mind of the person.*

Getting the mentals of a case is most difficult job, many times
it is impossible, *'patient's kuch batate hi nahi hai'*. The reality is,
if one develops his personal skill and takes keen interest in the job
soon it becomes the easiest job for him.

It is difficult to get mentals from children. In fact, through
their mannerisms in the physicians' chamber and from what parents
communicate through direct interaction, it often becomes easy to
get mentals of children who are much more open than elders and
speak out whatever is felt by them if a good communication is
established.

It is very difficult to know the mentals in illiterate people and
people from lower socio-economic strata. Infact these people have
intense emotions, greater conflicts, grief, deep-seated sentiments,
and complicated life situations and mental problems They are
highly charged emotional people although their sentiments may
be raw, coarse, it is for the physician to establish a rapport and get
symptoms from them. A right handling and right attitude in dealing
with them can bring the most characteristic mental picture. They
too are humans like all others and harbour same emotions. When
an illiterate rickshaw puller or a labourer opens his heart before
his close friend after a few pegs of country liquor it very much
signifies that he is an emotional person. You have to search the
way to the heart of these people, that really holds the key to
successful mental investigation.

Male patients rarely convey personal things to female
physicians and vice versa. A physician through his good
mannerisms, clarity of mind, pure conscience, decent behaviour
should be able to secure his patients confidence irrespective of
sex, age, caste, creed of his patient.

WHAT TO INVESTIGATE IN PATIENT'S MIND?

THE MENTAL STATE

The mental state is constituted in four things-**intellect, emotion, behaviour and functioning.**

Intellect

Under this we need to assess person's intelligence, comprehension, memory, perception, motivation, formulations of idea, thought concepts, discrimination and action -volition in the direction of choice conscience, level of confidence, will, as also the aberrations of perception and formulation i.e. delusion, illusion and hallucination, confusion, indecision etc.

Emotions

We need to know the basic emotions in the patient, those that are most marked, that influence his behaviour and his responses to the environment. Here it is important to judge the impulses guilt complex. The basic 'feeling state' responsible for the behavioural pattern must be taken into consideration while determining the remedy.

Behaviour

Behaviour, as our stalwarts define is the formalization of certain responses in a sequential manner or in short a reaction to the situation. The manner in which one behaves-aggressive, arrogant, mild, etc. should be very important to know the mind of the person and to deduce the mental state responsible for the behaviour.

Functioning

It is the manner in which he functions, example hard working, indolent, active or the manner in which he operates.

THE MENTAL EXPRESSIONS

It is also important that we know the patient's *expressions* in the form of anxiety, fear, grief, disappointment, frustration, anger, hatred, etc. But just knowing them isn't all important. Common emotions expressed in intense manner and peculiarities are of value here. We must also evaluate the cause, effect relationship between this, what leads to what, what comes first and what later, we need to understand the manner in which they have evolved in the patient. That is most important for us because anger is present in many drugs so is the anxiety so we need to find out the cause of his anger.

High Grade Mentals

According to Dr. Kent—fears, impulsive behaviour, perversions of instinct of survival like suicide and suicidal tendencies are considered high grade mentals. Again PQRS symptoms, the causative emotional factors, aggravating mentals, and concomitants also are high-grade mentals.

His temperament

According to Dr. Roberts the mental and emotional tendencies in reaction to time and environment, constitutes the temperament. Unless we know the temperament we cannot really know the individual.

Knowing the Real Mind

According to Dr. M.L. Dhawale—What one should be interested in is the evidence that leads us to a rational interpretation of:

Direct expressions: Like thought, perception, memory changes lack of will, indecisiveness, lowered competence, inappropriate activities etc.

Indirect expressions: The original emotions evoke strong feeling of guilt and this prevent direct expression and hence the subject takes on an exact opposite attitude.

Disturbed functioning: To voluntary autonomic nervous system and endocrinal system.

Dreams: Reflect unconscious drives and aspirations, anxiety and conflict at the subconscious level.

Dr. Kent says we do not know half as much about human mind as we think we do, we only know its manifestations. As per Dr. Dhawale we have to observe the activity in the person its presence, degree, absence, appropriateness to circumstance, its effect on self and degree of satisfaction. It is important for a physician to know, how has been the life of his patient in different phases right from childhood, adolescence, adult hood before and after marriage. His relations with people around, the circumstances in which he behaved in a particular manner, his feelings, his experience, the love or rejection he received from the environment.

INVESTIGATION

Human mind is complex and deep, human nature is varied, human behaviour is strange and unpredictable and human tendencies are devious and to investigate a mind certainly there is nothing so important than a detailed history, rather a detailed life story of the patient, which should be regarded as the first step. The next step is the interpretation of human mind from the available life story. It is important to identify the individual behind the life space written on the case paper and for this a case should be carefully worked out.

Knowing the mind of a person is not a simple affair never the less, it is neither too complex. Just a methodological approach is important if we want to investigate a patient's mind. If we want to know him as a person.

It involves following steps,

1. Recording patient's life story.

2. Analysis, evaluation and logical interpretation of this by the physician.

3. Physician's observation.

4. Information from the relatives and friends of the patient.

PREPARING THE PATIENT FOR INTERVIEW-PATIENT GUIDANCE AND EDUCATION

Only can a physician collect the relevant personal details from a patient if he is been able to win his faith and confidence. It is very important, that a physician thoroughly explain to the patient as—why his personal information especially at mental plane is needed. He should communicate it to him what importance does it hold in the patient's treatment. A physician should prepare a patient from this point of view. He should be told that history taking is a simple affair.

He may supply him with a pamphlet informing him in a simple yet convincing manner as to why and what information he needs. He has to effectively convey to him that if he shares the right information with the physician there are greater chances of his being cured. It should be straight away told to him that by telling right or wrong he will decide a cure for himself and thus ultimately his getting well is in his own hands. The patient's very first meeting with the physician is significant and it should leave a very good impression on the patient.

TYPES OF PATIENTS

1. Patients who carry their heart on their sleeves and extremely emotional will give out everything to the physician.

2. Intellectual parents who are shy and deceptive and will try to project false image revealing only 30 to 40 % of their self and hiding the rest.

3. Intelligent but plain persons will reveal upto 60 to 70% of information and hide what they want to. Never the less nobody will shares 100% information.

TYPES OF PHYSICIANS

1. Unprejudiced and skilled but beclouded with images of materia medica.

2. Prejudiced who carry firm fixed opinions about the male and female species in particular and people in general 'people are just like that type.'

3. Unprejudiced neither clouded but who are just psychoanalysts and lack the personal touch and end up being mechanical.

4. Slightly prejudiced with opinions about people in general yet who take a balanced view of everything and are able to establish a good rapport with the patient. These physicians can derive the maximum information from the patients.

BEFORE THE INTERVIEW

THE PHYSICIAN

As Dr. Roberts says the physician's attitude should be of rest and poise and he should not have any preconceived notions about the patient or his illness. It should be a quit listening attitude. The physician should himself be in a state of health. Mentally sound and stable. He should not be disturbed over anything, neither in a hurry. Because he is there not just to record the case but also to judge the person infront of him. He should enter into history taking with a positive frame of mind positively reassuring himself that he will get 'something' about the patient. The process involves observation, analysis, evaluation, logical interpretation, and finally synthesis so that a picture is finally resolved. A physician must be first a good psychologist.

As Dr. Dhawale guides us, a physician should be curious and genuinely interested in understanding his patient as a person. It is with this sole aim that he should go ahead with recording the history. He should himself relieve his anxieties about cure and whether or not will he be able to secure relevant information from the patient. All this enable a physician to reach the core of the patient and establish intimate patient physician's relationship. He should not inquire in a formal abrupt manner leading to a tense atmosphere preventing the patient to open up in front of the physician. So a physician has to be a normal, natural, himself. He should maintain a perfectly neutral attitude. He should not get emotionally involved. He should be a quiet listener who is able to establish a proper communication with patient. A sympathetic touch can do great miracles. Getting on with people is an art, which one develops out of the inherent interest in people. It should be an informal chat.

THE INTERVIEW

Dr. Dhawle's warning words the first and foremost thing a physician has to keep in mind is that the interview should not be too long and tiring for the patient. The physician should not try to drill too deep in the patient life, which may be offending for the patient. Delicacy and gentleness should be the two big mantras. The greatest success lies with the physician who is able to establish confidence in the patient. The patient should know you as the right person with whom he can share his personal information without hesitation. You have to use personal skill to establish rapport with the patient. The interview should not be a forceful interrogation but a gentle investigation. It should be rather a social interaction, a human-to-human dealing. It shouldn't be a question answer session but a casual chat where the physician speaks less and the patient more. Most of the times quiet listening with intermittent questions works well. The physician by placing tactful questions should get the patient talking and tactfully keep him talking without interfering, unless he drifts away. Try to reduce the gap between the two ends of the table make the patient comfortable. Establishing a comfort zone between him and you is very important. Do call elderly people uncle, aunty, dada, dadi, try to be a little informal and more social with them.

Whether leading questions should be asked ?

Yes, for confirmation of certain thing or to get the patients answers more precisely leading questions may be asked. But basically they must be avoided.

KICK STARTING

You should know how to handle people. For instance if a political leader comes to you, you may start your conversation with, 'You must be having a great hold in your party' and soon he will start to unwind himself before you. If he is a businessman you may commence 'these days its really difficult to carry on a business'. If she is a housewife you may initiate the conversation with a sympathizing statement, 'A housewife a housewife's job must be really strenuous and around the clock yet a thankless one.' With an old man you may begin the following manner, 'yours must have been a life full of varied colours, you must have seen everything in your life.'

Kick starting the patient is so important that kick plays the key otherwise a huge block obstructs the entire undertaking.

The art of listening and observation need to be cultivated. The physician needs to cash on the very thing that once triggered, everyone is interested and eager to talk about oneself, so is the patient. The patient is very much interested in pouring out his complaints to the sympathetic physician who lends his ear. You have to bring the patient to that dynamism where he tells everything about him. You have to bring him to a stage where he is excited and spills the beans easily. Going along the line of patient's dreams may be helpful in many cases. The physician has to bring the patient close to himself. He has to bring him close to his understanding of self.

The question's wordings should be simple and unambiguous. As all of us know they should not give any hint or should not be suggestive. The choice of the word should be according to the level of intelligence of the patient. The physician must be very particular in noting the very expressions of the patient in his language, which may help him in interpretation later on. The patient should be asked about his mood on the very day and feeling state in last few days. Always keep in mind that it is just one colour that the patient wears before you. Trust but also suspect your patient. Trust him first don't indulge in suspicion, for suspicion, may erode your entire judgment. Try to keep a balance between suspicion and trust. We must keep track of our patient throughout the treatment, observe him in days to come, his behaviour, his demands from you as it can give a fair idea to the physician about the patient. A physician must read the patient eyes which never hide the reality.

Suspect those patients where you feel the information has come out more easily than you expected too. Such patients may seem to have opened their heart before you but in reality they may have taken you for a ride. Assess whether the patient is telling the truth or is he just wants to 'finish the job'. Also judge whether a patient while telling about himself is entering into his fantasies or bluffing. Second look is very important, looking at it entirely through a different angle is important. Knowledge and experience of human nature hold the key in your interpretations. The physician's insight is important. He must catch the attitude.

INTELLIGENT PHYSICIAN AND SKILLED INTERROGATION

Right from the moment the patient enter the physician's chamber his work of understanding him as a person begins. Roberts says that the mental symptoms should be observed from the attitude of the patient. Every one carries an attitude with him. As the patient is busy telling a mental symptoms the physician should try to keep his focus on that particular symptom.

Patient's movement and expression should be watched. His posture, dress, carriage, behaviour convey many things about him. His hesitation, ego, arrogance, confidence etc. have to be observed and noted. As Dr. Hahnemann recommends—Observe the 'altered and unusual' character about him. Make a note of it, if he appears, quarrelsome, in haste, anxious, sad, depressed, dull. How was his comprehension of the questions asked to him and responses, tone coherence, eye expressions. His responses indicate his alertness, intellect, mental susceptibility, which is important for the physician.

In the Organon of medicine Dr. Hahnemann has stressed that the state of mind and disposition is what the physician has to observe during clinical trial.

He has to be an attentive observer and fidelity in tracing the picture of the disease is important. He has to observe not see, listen not just hear and smell the air around the patient.

Dr. Dhawale says, more attention should be paid on 'How it is said' rather than what is said. The changes in the expression of the patient while describing some things should be taken a note of. There are moments during the case history where the patient is just 'himself.' The physician should take a careful note of them. He should base his interpretations accordingly. The body language needs to be watched.

According to Dr. Dhawale, during the interview it becomes obvious that he is deliberately avoiding reference to certain issues by side tracking them. The physician has to make a strong note of it and investigate and explore them in future visits. If the patient seems unwilling to tell things about himself do not dig much further other wise he will get irritated. The physician should promote spontaneity on part of the patient. The different replies to the same question put in different context and altering words the replies enable us to determine to what extent the patient is a reliable observer.

Dr. Hahnemann says hysterical patient should be carefully interrogated. Such patients tell their complaints in an exaggerated manner. Ask a sudden intelligent question and catch him unaware and involuntarily the truth comes out. Here the first spontaneous reactions have to be specially noted although the patient may deny it at the next instance.

We have to be aware of those who are expert in language and use it rather to conceal the thoughts than to reveal, they often take you for a good round. One of my patient took me to such a long ride I labelled him Phosphorus when in reality he was a Calcarea. What is left unsaid and untouched by the patient is most important. No response from the patient on a particular matter itself is a suggestive response and should be rightly interpreted. Many a times you may get the 'few clues' like ' I don't tell anything to anyone, may he be a doctor or a lawyer,' revealing that the patient is a secretive individual.

RELIABILITY OF DATA- DOES IT AFFECT OUR WORK ?

Never access a patient on his face value, basically you must trust your patient first then suspect. He may or may not have provided you the right information. In homeopathy too, the case value is more important than the face value. Whether a patient provides true information or false information we must remember that the real self cannot be hidden it slips out. His self gets expressed whether or not he gives true information. A physician does not judge the patient merely from the information that the patient provides to the physician but the judgment is on the interpretation of the information on the ground of evidences, in the patient's life story.

It should be so swiftly and softly done that neither the patient realizes that he has shared his entire life story with the physician nor does he feels that the physician has gone in so depth in the patients life history. It should be a smart affair. Ultimately it depends on the successful content blow the physician is the patient.

Interpretating the patient's story—On what is it based ?

* Exact observation.

* Logical interpretation.

* Scientific corrélation.

* Rational explanation.

How is it done?

1. You have to make columns: Phase, Situation, Reaction, Interpretation and Reason. Put the patient's information and try to judge why a patient behaved in a particular manner in a particular situation. You must try to find out the cause the reason behind a patient's reaction in a particular situation. 'Why' he reacted in the particular way should lead you to his

mental state. You must note your interpretation and the grounds for it.

2. Where you find everything 'goody goody' in patient's life space with the patient expressing that he has 'no problems,' that means things are exactly reverse of what they seem.

3. Look for the missing links in the data. Look for the lacunas.

4. Two statements of the patient may contradict each other on one hand he may say I am a philanthropist and on other hand some of his responses may express a greed for money.

5. Use inductive and deductive logic.

6. A conclusion needs to be drawn under a particular circumstances by which the patient is judged accordingly.

SOME KEY INQUIRIES

Inquiry about father and mother's nature and habits, also the nature, habits tendencies of siblings helps us to identify genetic traits in the family and the child also. It also helps in understanding the nature of the person. This is useful especially in children who are too young to convey anything. Again traits in certain communities (community traits) classes (class traits) and area traits should be useful to a physician in understanding the patient of that particular community, class or area etc.

In recording the history remember 'if your patient gives you an inch, you should take an yell,' in certain areas.

Personal secretes can be revealed by skillful framing of questions. Never get disappointed if you don't get details and patient seems to be uncooperative in the first visit. In visits to come, he may convey you everything. May be on future occasions he should be with his real natural self and in a good mood to express out things. The physician's correct interpretation is all that matters at the end. A patient may be told to prepare a write up for he may feel more free to write than verbally communicate to you. While writing he may recollect many things about himself than when instantaneously asked. It also gives a good chance to the physician to check, confirm information and look for the missing links.

SOME SPECIALLY DESIGNED QUESTIONS FOR CHILDREN
(HERE A GIRL CHILD IS CONSIDERED)

1. How is your child ?

2. How is her activity, play etc ?

3. Does she share her objects ?

4. How does she keeps her toys, books and other things ?

5. If her demands are not fulfilled how does she react?

6. How does she react to when shouted at ?

7. How is her reaction to parental fights ?

8. How is her behaviour at school ?

9. What does the teacher say about her?

10. Behaviour at home with family members, friends, strangers?

11. How is her performance at school in studies and other activities ?

12. What are her likings- toys, friends, playing, reading etc.?

13. Does she fear some things ?

14. Is she weepy? And off and on tends to get irritable?

15. Has she witnessed the death of any family member if yes her response during that period?

16. Her favourite subjects in study ?

17. How is she during the exam period?

Besides inquiry with the parents, the physician should try to establish a friendly contact with the child and try to get an idea about him. He should also closely observe his activities in the clinic. Ask him about his friends about dreams and his likings etc.

QUESTIONS FOR ADULTS

1. How is your nature?

2. How are your relations presently with your family members and associates?

3. How do you deal with the tensions and problems at work?

4. Have they affected your health?

5. Do you enjoy being alone or like to be with people?

6. How was your Childhood? Were your needs then fulfilled?

7. How was your youth?

8. Any pink spots?

9. How is your married life?

10. Has there been any change in your nature life now and then or after marriage?

11. What have been the major milestones in your life?

12. Attachments? Have they fulfilled your expectations?

13. Any memorable incident that has left an impact on you/ that you remember often?

14. Have you ever been sad/depressed or happy/elated? Are there any change of moods? When things don't happen as per your

wishes how do you react? How do you express your anger or displeasure?

15. If you listen anybody speaking badly about you or playing behind the back games what do you do?

16. How do you deal with people who are not in good terms with you or jealous?

17. What are your ambitions and are they fulfilled?

18. What is important for you name, fame or money or recognitions?

19. Do you consider yourself successful in life?

20. What are you looking forward to in your life?

21. What do you feel about it?

22. How do you think is your ability to take decisions or work for long hours?

23. How is your ability to concentrate or study for long time?

24. Your performance in studies and other activities?

25. Are you nervous before undertaking a work, examination meeting or a programme? How much?

26. What do you feel like doing things from bottom of your heart and which gives you real happiness?

27. Do you suppress your thoughts/feelings?

28. What do family members and people say about you?

29. Describe yourself in three to four words?

STUDY OF THE MIND OF A DRUG AND THE PATIENT

- Basic mental state.

- Intensity of symptoms.

- The characteristic, peculiar, mental symptoms.

- Queer, rare, strange mentals.

- Mental evolution (development).

- Manner in which mental expressions develop.

- Their connection, relation, arrangement.

- That 'what leads to what, i.e. the cause effect relationship between these expressions.

- Thus the 'life history', the 'mental story' of this patient.

CHAPTER 8

THE CORRECT CONSTITUTIONAL PRESCRIBING

A physician should skillfully secure all the relevant information from the patient to make a correct prescription. If he proceeds for recording the history of the patient in the following manner, his half job is already done. A case well recorded is half cured. A detailed case history facilitates a physician to select a right remedy. For this it is important that the case should be recorded 'intellectually'. The inquiry should be made in such a manner that its outcome is the 'picture of the patient,' and not merely the information. For this it is important that the physician frames his questions based on certain points and a detailed history should becomes easily available to him.

THE HISTORY

The history to begin with should include all the basic things name, age sex, address, marital status, vegetarian or non-vegetarian, age of marriage.

PARTICULARS OF THE PATIENT

Age:

Sex:

Status:

Age of marriage:

Education:

Religion:

Occupation: The nature of work, stresses- mental, physical.

Local complete address with phone number:

Patient address helps in telling in knowing the environment he lives and may point to certain causative or exciting factors or continuous exposure.

PARTICULARS OF THE FAMILY MEMBERS

Details of the family members should be recorded as they give an idea about the 'background' of the patient.

Father: Name, Age, Education, Occupation.

Mother: —do—

Spouse: ——do—

Sibling: M/F- Name, Age, Class.

Children: M/F-Age.

CHIEF COMPLAINT

This should be recorded considering the following points

Duration, Causation, Modalities, Sensations, Concomitants, Location, Extension.

MODALITIES

Positional modalities.

Seasonal modalities.

Thermal modalities.

Time modalities.

Sweat aggravation, amelioration.

Sleep aggravation, amelioration.

Emotional modalities.

Other Modalities

Sensitivity, light, sound, touch, odor, food, and drink, moon Phases, thought- thinking of complaints.

Concomitants

Fever, thermal reaction, desire for covers, thirst, appetite, sleep, mentals- irritable, dull, weak. These are immensely helpful in selecting a remedy and often concise the choice of a simillimum. The auxiliary symptoms combine with the chief complaints to give you a picture of the remedy.

The chief complaint must be carefully recorded because it is the complaint where the patient as a person will get expressed. According to Dr. Herbert Roberts 'the chief complaint has a psychological value of maximum proportion in homeopathic prescribing. It brings the patient to the physician and if the physician responds by careful questioning he can draws out the history of other symptoms and the patient feels a satisfaction and confidence that the physician is not treating his case as of no consequence."

Associated Complaints

Every associated complaint must also be recorded under the above heads.

PATIENT AS A PERSON

General appearance: Height, Weight:

Appetite:

Here the complete schedule of all meals other feeds should be recorded so that one gets the correct idea about the appetite of the person.

Thirst:

Quantity of water, frequency, particular timings, quality of water (Cold, Luke warm, Normal).

Addictions:

Tobacco, tea, coffee, alcohol etc.

Pica:

Desire for chalk, clay, sand, wall lime, slate pencils coal, or unusual things, indigestible things, odor/fumes of petrol, diesel.

Disordered by:

Fats, cold food, non-veg, starches etc.

Desires and Aversion:

Sweet, sour, spicy, simple, salty, milk, ghee, butter, fruits, hot cold food, other specific food items.

Discharges

1. Stool:

Frequency, quantity, character, complaints before during and after EG pain, burning, pain in abdomen, tenesmus etc worms, itch.

Urine:

Perspiration:

Quantity, parts, odor, stains

Sex function:

Sexual desire, frequency, satisfaction, masturbation, premarital, extramarital, prostitution.

Complaints during and after coition like backache, urinary complaints etc other related things guilt, impotency, fear, aversion.

FEMALE (FOR FEMALE PATIENTS)

Menses:

Menarche, last menstrual period, cycles: regular, irregular, days/duration.

Character: Colour, odor, quantity, clots, stains.

Complaints: Before menses, during menses, after menses,

Menopause and related complains.

Past History:

Changes in cycle after delivery, marriage or any other milestone.

Modalities (at what time of the day is it more).

Causation: Emotions, suppression- foot wetting, mental sufferings.

Leucorrhoea:

Character: Thick, thin, profuse, scanty, color, odor, stains.

Sensations: Itching, irritating, burning, modalities, accompaniments relation with menstruation.

Pregnancy:

Nature, complaints, pica, mental state.

Abortions:

Type, period, complications.

Lactation.

Lochia.

FOR CHILDREN

Mother's Gestation notes

Complaint and disorders of mother during pregnancy.

Pica, mental state and environment during pregnancy, time of conception, whether a welcome child.

Birth notes: Term- full term or premature, nature of delivery- cesarean, normal, forceps, labour- obstructed, cry- Normal or delayed, post-partum complains and complications, neonatal diseases.

Birth weight.: In Lbs.

Breast feeding: Details, till how many months.

Weaning: Month, foods, acceptance.

Vaccination: BCG: Birth 3 Days.

DPT/Oral ½ M

———————— 2½ M

———————— 3½ M

Measles: 9 month

DPT/Oral Boo.1 ½ Yr.

TYP/TET: 5-6 Yr

Development

I. Physical:

Head holding: 2-3 Months.

Turning: 5-6 months.

Sitting with support: 5-6 months.

Sitting without support: 7-8-9 month.

Crawling: 9-10 months.

Standing with support: 10 month.

Standing without support: 11-12 months.

Walking with support: 1 yr.

Walking without support: 1¼-1½ yr.

Dentition: 5-6 Months.

Speech: Monosyllable: 1Yr.

Jargons: 1¼4r.

Sentences: 1-3/4Yr.

II. Mental Development

Nature: Activity, play, beatings, fights, objects-sharing, keeping, demanding.

Behavior: School, family, friends, strangers.

Performance: School and other activities.

Likings: Toys, friends, play.

Expressions: Fear, mischievous.

Irritable, weepy.

Sensitivity: Parental fights, beating.

SLEEP AND DREAMS

Time, sound/disturbed, light/sensitive/deep/naps, refreshing /unrefreshing, symptoms during sleep-grinding/biting teeth, walking, talking, crying, moaning, perspiration, position, startling in sleep.

Dreams: Details. Persistent/Frequent, impact.

PHYSICAL REACTIONS

. Bathing, covers, food, season, fanning reactions —cloud, open air, change of weather, rainy weather, wet getting, exposure to drafts, sun heat, perspiration.

PAST HISTORY

Measles, chicken pox, whooping cough, pneumonia bronchitis, diphtheria, neo—asphyxia, jaundice etc.

FAMILY HISTORY

Mother: MGM, MGF, MA , MU.

Patient side: Paternal grand mother, grand father, Maternal side: Maternal grand mother, grand father, uncles/aunt, uncle/aunt, Sibling; M/F.

This should include acute and chronic diseases, even trivial complaints, operations, hereditary diseases, genetic defects, mentals especially of father and mother, tendencies to bleed, of delayed healing, to catch cold etc. Whether there has been blood relationship between their ancestors-consanguinity plays an important role in hereditary tendencies and also homeopathic selection.

PHYSICAL FINDINGS

Proceed organ wise from head to foot. Besides complete clinical examination look for spots on nails skins, any genetic defect, graying of hair, extra growth, cracks on palms, soles and other marked features.

TREAMENT HISTORY

This should include the details of all the previous treatments and investigations done.

TEMPERAMENT ASSESSMENT

The physician must be able to find out into which temperament his patient fits nervous, bilious, sanguinous and phlegmatic or whether a combination of the above. Temperament includes functional physiological tendencies of circulation, elimination, respiration and mental and emotional tendencies in reaction to environment and circumstances.

Investigating the mentals- Kindly refer the previous chapter.

SOME KEY INQUIRIES

Inquiry about father and mother's nature and habits also the habits of siblings helps us to identify genetic traits in the family and the child also.

This is useful especially in children who are too young and in whom collection of mental is a difficult task. Again traits in certain communities (community traits) classes (class traits) and area traits should be useful to a physician in understanding the patient of that particular community, class, area etc.

CONSTITUTIONAL PRESCRIBING: THE ENIGMA REVEALED

IST STEP: CONSTRUCTING THE TOTALITY

Master Hahnemann has mentioned in aphorism 7 once totality is sketched the most difficult task is accomplished. Totality of symptoms is nothing but the uncommon, characteristic, peculiar symptoms of the patient arranged in a logical order so as to construct the image of the patient. As per Dr. K. N. Kasad, "Totality is an idea, a concept a mental abstraction which we conceptualize from the available facts (case history). Its construction involves logical interpretation of symptoms/data by a physician guided by philosophy."

For constructing a totality one should first diagnose the case correctly. After one arrives at the diagnosis the uncommon characteristic symptoms of the patient must be separated from the common symptoms of the disease. Dr. Roberts stresses, 'we must not fail to recognize the value of the totality of the symptoms and this must take into consideration the chief complaints, those of which the patient most often complaints plus the peculiar characteristics of the patient. If both these elements are present, we may be sure we are on the right track' (to cure).

These are the symptoms, which denote the individual response of the person to the environment. Next these 'personal symptoms' are evaluated i.e. placed in the order of importance. The evaluation of Kent, Boenninghausen and Boger and other pioneers should be considered.

Symptoms should be first analyzed into generals and characteristic particulars. The generals should be differentiated into mental generals, physical generals and pathological generals. Every symptom both general as well as a characteristic particular should be differentiated into causation, modalities, sensation and concomitant and location arranged respectively according to importance. (Kindly refer the Fig.3) Only then it will be regarded a complete symptom. This logical arrangement of the symptoms in the proper order constitutes totality.

Totality should be constructed over the total period of time over which the phenomenon of disease occurs. The roots of the disease may be traced backwards to the past and prognosticated forwards. Only the present state of the disease can never constitute a proper totality. " Dr. Hahnemann in Aphorism 3 has mentioned if the physician clearly perceives what is to be cured in the diseases that is to say in every individual case of the disease, if he clearly perceives what is curative in medicines, that is to say in each individual medicine and if he knows how to adapt, according to clearly defined principles what is curative in medicines to be undoubtedly morbid in the patient, so that recovery must ensue. Hence for a true homeopathic physician only knowledge about medicines won't accomplish the study of the science but it is the study of the patient and his ailment from an individualistic viewpoint and for this the proper construction of totality -the individual image is very essential. While constituting the totality the portrait of the patient should be essentially sketched. If this is not done it clearly reveals that a totality is just mechanically made. The totality should reflect the mind, the person as a whole, to the physician who has made it.

TOTALITY OF SYMPTOMS

1. General Symptoms :   a)   Mental Generals
                          b)   Physical Generals
                          c)   Pathological Generals
   (further division as that of characteristic particulars
   given below)
2. Characteristic Particulars-
   a) Causation –Mental and physical
   b) Modalities –Aggravation and Amelioration-Mental
                                                      Physical
   c) Sensation
   d) Concomitant- Mental
                           Physical
   e) Location

Ideal Totality

This should include the symptoms under the following heads:

Generals followed by Particulars

Causation

Modalities

Sensation

Concomitants

Location

But practically the totality where information regarding many of the above is missing may be constituted in the following:

Practical totality

Generals followed by Particulars

   Causation+ Sensation

Causation+Location

Sensation + Location

Concomitant + sensation

Causation+ Concomitant

Any of the above combination.

IIND STEP: ROLE OF REPERTORIZATION IN PRESCRIBING

Repertorization to most is merely a mathematical process, which brings forth the indicated remedy for the patient. A common idea about repertorization is considering the symptoms of the patient, finding the appropriate rubrics for the same, repertorizing the case and considering the remedy having the highest marks and covering maximum rubrics, to be the simillimum for the case. By no means is repertorization a direct mathematical and easy process of selecting a simillimum. By repertorization we only arrive at a group of the possible remedies indicated for the case. Repertory by no means is an end in itself but it is a means, which makes selection of simillimum easy. For final selection of the simillimum we must look into Materia Medica compare the patient's image with that of the resulting drugs and then chose a similar remedy.

The result of repertorization only indicates to us the remedies that are likely to 'go close' to the patient. A remedy with lesser number of marks may be finally selected as the simillimum. On the other hand a remedy scoring the highest marks and covering most of rubrics of the case may not be the final remedy of the patient, if it doesn't resemble the 'portrait' of the patient. The selection of homeopathic remedy is based on a qualitative and not on a quantitative evaluation. Homeopathic therapeutics is based on fixed principles and essentially qualitative and hence it demands a qualitative approach to every aspect including the repertorization.

REPERTORIZATION

PHILOSOPHY

Before repertorization the first thing that one has to thoroughly understand is the philosophy of different repertories and then only he can make the choice of repertory needed for his case. It is very essential for a physician to read the introduction and preface to the repertories and also the philosophical background instead of directly proceeding for the repertory proper. If proper repertory is selected considering the background of its philosophy it can give handy aid in selecting simillimum. For instance in a case with predominant mentals Kent's repertory will be most appropriate. A large separate chapter dealing with mind with well verified symptoms finds place in the Kent's repertory. In a case with pathological generals Boger's repertory will be suitable considering its philosophical background. Thus knowing the philosophical background is very essential for selection of a repertory for a given case.

MAKING THE REPERTORIAL TOTALITY

The next step is forming the repertorial totality. For this the understanding of the fundamentals of repertorization is very essential. The basic principle of repertorization is to proceed from generals to particulars. Hence we must proceed from generals to particulars. The generals should be considered in the first phase of the repertorization, while the reportorial totality is made and in the final phase. We must consider the peculiar, queer, rare, and strange symptoms of the patient, the characteristic particulars with characteristic modalities which point to a fewer remedies. It is essentially important that the remedies covering the generals of the patient(and thus the patient) are not left out hence we proceed in this manner.

Dr. Hahnemann says, 'Write out all the mental symptoms and all symptoms predicated of the patient himself and search the repertory for the symptoms that correspond to these'. The generals include mental generals, general aggravations and ameliorations, physical generals like desire for peculiar things, thirst appetite, sleep etc. It should be noted that the circumstances that makes a whole being feel better or worse are of greater importance than when the same circumstance only affects particular part. While making a reportorial totality only the uncommon, peculiar characteristic symptoms of symptoms of the patient must be considered. Common symptoms like headache, weakness, diarrhoea assume no importance & should not be considered. If these symptoms are considered, a vast number of insignificant remedies will prominently emerge after repertorization none of which will be close to the patient. The successful use of any repertory depends heavily upon the physician's skillful perception of valuable symptom in a given case. The reportorial totality with the 'Prized symptoms' should construct an image of the patient to the physician.

SELECTING THE CORRECT CONSTITUTIONAL REMEDY

One must first study the range of remedies that come to your mind (or are the result of repertorization) after you have recorded and analyzed a case, and prepared the totality. If no remedy seems to go closer with the patient then pick up two/three peculiarities of the case and study the remedies which carry them. See if the other symptoms of the remedy, match with the patient. Dr. Kent says 'Use a key to examine the remedy and see if it has all the other symptoms that the patient has.'

Like patients our remedies too are deceptive and sly and a remedy at first reading or consideration may not seem to match with the patient but on further study, reading and comparing it will be revealed that it goes 'very close' to the patient. So the core of the remedy, the 'inner self' of the remedy should match with that of the patient. Repeated study of the remedies, disclose many key things about them to us.

If no remedy matches the patient as a whole, prescribe a remedy that runs close with generals of the patient and has marked action on the organs affected (covers the chief and associated complaints also). The generals constitute the patient. In many cases at physical level, the characteristics are scanty. But there is a resemblance at mental level and with a few even two or three physical features (especially generals) matching with the patient the remedy can well be the simillimum for the case. Occasionally prescriptions are to be based only on the resemblance at the mental level. According to Dr. Roberts although Dr. Hahnemann stressed more on individual the peculiar characteristic signs and symptoms of the case but he never neglected other symptoms in making a prescription. He had the genius of giving each symptom its true place in the picture without distorting the totality. Hence we must adopt the golden mean between the two points—the general (vague) symptoms and individual symptoms to assure us of a true totality.

In many cases you may not get the exact features of remedies in materia medica, as in your patient. For example the patient may not tell you that his urine smells like a horse's urine but he may say its 'very very offensive' here you have to asses the intensity of his the odor correlate things and a remedy like Nitric acid may be indicated. If a particular section of the totality points to some few remedies examine them for general resemblance. The remedy may be right before your eyes.

A remedy should never be considered 'contra indicated' for example you cannot discard a remedy just because patient doesn't have one or two symptoms of the remedy. A remedy always has to be 'indicated' in homeopathy on the basis of marked resemblance. One should remember not to discard a remedy because it doesn't cover the 'remaining' symptoms of the patient. Quantity has no scope in homeopathy. It should cover the essence of the patient.

The key to finding the right remedy is to keep focus on the generals of the case and the uncommon, peculiar symptoms, leaving aside the common symptoms. The physician should try to locate the 'patient' in the entire history, which may be compounded in three or four peculiarities. That's really important for a perfect prescription. And rest symptoms in a case remain as insignificant as a scrap.

By a deep study of the patient's totality you may be able to recognize to which group the peculiarities of the patient belong for example: Natrum group, Calcarea group etc. and then you should look and study the individual remedies of the group and see which one goes most close to the patient.

Homeopathy is no mathematics where one plus one is essentially two. In homeopathy it can be four five or even six. Homeopathy is simple and simply excellent. There are no fixed criteria or rigid rules for prescribing although some principles, and considerations are worked upon on the basis of homeopathic philosophy. The approach to a case should be scientific and the resultant should be a good prescription underlying some logic. A physician when selecting a particular remedy should have substantial ground on which he selects the particular remedy. He should himself know the reason why he has selected a remedy. He should himself be convinced over the selection.

Differentiating a scientist from an artist Dr. Stuart Close says 'A scientist on the contrary never, or rarely, proceeds by instinct. His eyes are open from the beginning. He knows what to do. Reason and logic, rather than feeling and emotion, are his guides from first to last.'

He expresses that homeopathy is both an art and a science. The successful homeopathic must be both an artist and a scientist. His work must be both artistic and scientific. Technique must be governed by definite principles.

In prescribing it ultimately comes to prescribing on physician's individual logic, intelligence, skill, knowledge, the images of remedies in his mind and most importantly his homeopathic philosophical depth. You have to simply get the patient in the available data. You may get him there in the mentals greatly resembling a particular remedy or he may be there in the physicals of a case resembling another. You have to 'catch him' with your knowledge mimicking a remedy. He ought to simulate some remedy, which is writing on the rock.

Your mind should capture him. 'There he is' should be the response of the mind when, the remedy resembling your patient is being studied by you. Everything in the patient and the remedy cannot be similar. Resemblance weakens at some level. But throughout the spirit of the remedy should match with the spirit of the patient. Heart of the remedy should be matched with the heart of the patient. And you should be sure at heart about this resemblance.

But in many cases there may be a marked resemblance in entirety and the patient may resemble the remedy at all the three levels greatly (Mental generals, physical generals and characteristic particulars) and also a strong resemblance in the miasmatic background may be there. This is an ideal simillimum.

In the final selection of the remedy the miasmatic background should be given preference over the thermality. And the points in totality (refer fig 3) should be given importance in the order they are arranged in the totality.

A physician must look if the 'personality' of the drug matches with the personality of the patient. For this the images of the chronic remedies should be well sketched in his mind, this is the most significant aspect of correct prescribing. Mind has to be properly fed with the images of the remedies. And then a selection of a constitutional remedy may be made even in minutes and even without the help of repertorization. Through proper mental training and mending your mind you should be able to instantaneously recognize 'him' in your patient- the 'Natrum' the 'Calcarea' the 'Kali' etc.

A 'patient' may be present in any 'section' in a case.

The patient may well be hidden in any of the following:

1. One uncommon characteristic peculiar symptom+ Few marked generals mental or physical.

2. Few Characteristic particulars + Mental generals.

3. Just two or three un common peculiar symptoms. (Which may be generals or characteristic particulars.)

4. Simply the Mental generals.

5. Simply the Physical generals.

If a remedy is selected scientifically and logically any number of physicians should select the same remedy as the simillimum for the patient. The key to correct prescription lies in the correct appreciation of the patient's image. You have to hold your patient infront of the mirror of materia medica and the image of the remedy will be before your eyes. Homeopathy is drawing a straight line between the two points the remedy and the patient. To conclude I would like to quote Dr. G Srinivasulu Homeopathy is a simple 'Match the following'. Always remember science never fails but it is we humans who falter, there are no lacunas in a science but sure something may be lacking in us. So we need not blame our science for our failures, but locate our faults and try to improve.

CAUTION

Prevent yourself from the habit formation at mind that these particular remedies come for the 'particular affections'. We treat a patient with an individual remedy not the disease with particular remedies.

Dr. Robert's cautions 'Key notes often give us a clue to the indicated remedy, but the clue must not be allowed to overbalance our judgment in weighing the whole symptom picture.' Judgment of susceptibility is the key to everything in homeopathy.

An Ideal Prescription

- It should be a logical one.

- It should be based on homeopathic philosophy and not just the Materia medica.

- It should show full regard to the homeopathic principles laid down by the Master Hahnemann.

- It should prove the mantra *minimum medicine, maximum effect.*

- It should satisfy the medical conscience of the physician.

- It should make a physician confident of a sure cure ahead.

Although based on minimum symptoms it should be for the diseased individual and not for his disease.

Such a prescription surely promises a physician nothing but a DYNAMIC CURE.

CHAPTER 9

THE SUCCESSFUL SECOND PRESCRIPTION

Homeopathic philosophy and Kent's twelve observations give a lot of guidelines about a second prescription. As all of us know a second prescription may be a repetition of the first, a complementary medicine, an antidote, a change of remedy, or even a change of potency and it can be very well based on the guidelines of homeopathic philosophy. I don't wish to make the repetition of the same here. I wish to bring to notice and stress on some key points in this section. Through this chapter I wish to put focus on some significant points.

Normally in a chronic case you should expect a response in any form from the patient in fifteen to twenty days after the first prescription. You may wait for another week when you are very sure of the remedy you selected for the patient. We should give sufficient time for the remedy to act. Most of the times one may get a delayed response. Responses to an administered remedy are unpredictable and depend on the patients inherent susceptibility and susceptibility to the Simillimum and undoubtedly on your right selection. If the physician has been successful in perfectly satisfying the susceptibility of the patient with a 'Potential Simillimum' an early response is expected.

Some times we often get a delayed response even if the selected remedy and potency are correct. The nature of the disease has also a role to play. In the presence of gross pathologies and very long standing diseases, response is often slow. In acute and more superficial complaints response is quite fast. Here the seat of the disease should be considered. In deep seated diseases often a longer period is required for a response and in many cases repeated stimuli of medicine are needed.

Even in some chronic cases one may get a response to the simillimum in just few days but that should not be considered the final response, it should be observed over a period of time until the patient seems ameliorated for a considerable period. A response may well be received in a seven days time. In acute cases a response may be received in four/eight/twelve/twenty four or forty eight hours. A no change in acute emergencies definitely calls for a change of remedy but still a day or two may be given to the remedy.

KEY NOTES ON FOLLOW UP PRESCRIPTION
* Never be in a hurry to change the remedy.
* Do not change a remedy unless you have substantial and logical reasons.
* Do not hesitate to change the potency.
* A placebo may be the best second prescription under all circumstances.
* An indicated remedy is more likely to be the best antidote as well as the complementary.
* Never repeat when the patient is improving.
* Never change when Hering's law is being followed.
* Never change a remedy when a discharge or eruptions follows the administration.

They are so many factors influencing the action of the remedy on the patient so we must always give a second chance to a well selected remedy. One may get no response at all with the first dose. This by no means signifies that the remedy is not a correct one. It has to be given another chance to prove its similarity. Remedies need different time to act on different individuals of different sex, age, susceptibility. In chronic cases when you don't get a response to a well selected and things come to a standstill, you should think of a change of potency going to a higher potency. And even after the change of potency of the indicated remedy the disease draws its heads up, then it is the time to administer the anti-miasmatic remedy.

In cases of cough, acute skin troubles, itching etc., a patient may show no change for two days and then total amelioration. So it is necessary to give time to every remedy. Giving time and also a second chance is important.

Do not hurry or become restless try to see behind the disease expressions of the patient try to assess what is likely to happen. Look for the reduced congestion in throat and improvement in the generals of the patient even a better general look may guide you that cure is somewhere round the corner. If your selection is proper put full faith in your remedy and give it sufficient time to act. Some times hurry is likely to interfere with the possible action of the remedy. Worry draws hurry. Trust your science, your selection, do not worry.

A response or no response should always be judged under the light of philosophy. It should be an intellectual assessment and not an emotional judgment.

Remedies need time to act. And we need to give it to them. It may happen that you are just about to witness the wonderful curative effect of the remedy with the amelioration in the disease and you prescribe another remedy complicating the things and disturbing the action of the remedy. This should be avoided under all circumstances. Never repeat when the patient is improving.

Never change when Hering's law is being followed.

Never change a remedy when a discharge or eruptions follows the administration.

When we witness a medicinal aggravation we must first wait so that it comes down on its own. Now when selecting an antidote or the next remedy the question which may trouble the intelligent minds is that whether to consider the symptoms of the remedy in our 'next totality' or not. The answer is, yes we must consider these new symptoms and prescribe for the 'changed malady'.

Dr. kent says, 'The second prescription, then, technically speaking, is the prescription after the one that has acted. Consider the first prescription the one that has acted, that one has effected changes, and subsequent to that the next prescription is the second.'

As per Dr. Roberts, 'The reaction to correct prescription is that the striking features, the peculiar features, the concomitant symptoms on which the choice of the remedy was based are the first symptoms to be removed.'

The key to a successful second prescription is not the right selection of the prescription itself (i.e. the remedy) but assessing the real need of it. And rightly satisfying that need. The physician should try to judge whether it is really needed or not. For an intelligent skillful prescriber the most successful second prescription often is a placebo. As per the guidelines in Organon Dr Hahnemann says in acute cases a well indicated remedy should be given in medium potency first and the effect of each dose repeated after two three hours should be watched. If improvement is seen the remedy should be stopped or at least the interval between doses be lengthened. In case of no improvement reconsider the case, see if the totality points to another remedy, if not repeat the first chosen drug and preferably in a higher potency the remedy should be reconsidered. In chronic cases, case should be reviewed from time to time. If improvement ceases a remedy should be repeated in same potency if still no further improvement is seen potency should be increased. If still no improvement is seen an intercurrent remedy should be given.

I would like to conclude this section with Dr. Kent's concluding paragraph. " No prescription can be made for any patient except after a careful and prolonged study of the case, to know what it promises in the symptoms, and everything that has existed previously. That is the important thing. Always restudy the cases. Do not administer a medicine without knowing the constitution of the patient, because it is a hazardous and dangerous thing to do".

■

CHAPTER 10

TELEPHONIC PRESCRIBING

Often a physician has to prescribe a remedy over telephone especially when managing out of station patients. Many a times when the patient himself is unable to personally come to a physician's clinic the physician has to base his prescription on the telephonic conversation with the patient. And this really needs a skill. Here the 'telephonic conversation' is the only totality on which he has to base his selection. The intelligence and logic of the physician is at real test when he is needed to prescribe on the basis of his electronic communication with the patient without actually seeing and examining him. Primarily it is advisable not to prescribe a medicine over telephone without actually seeing the patient. But under certain circumstances the physician may be needed to do this.

Basics

- Strong imagination.
- Skilled questioning.
- Precise correlation.
- Intelligent 'listening', and not just 'hearing.'
  hold the key.
- Getting the 'sense' of the verbal expression.

The physician needs to be in a clear mindset and all his senses of perception need to be alert and ready. The physician must keep a paper and pen in the hand and note down his entire communication with the patient in the words of the patient.

HOW TO GO AHEAD WITH IT?

The first and foremost thing a physician should ask the patient is to 'describe in details' his present complaints. The physician is expected not to miss on the minute details, which the patient verbally conveys to him.

The voice of the patient holds everything 'What does he tell first? What does he start with ? What's his main suffering? What is greatly troubling him? This first needs to be focused while making a prescription. It should be given prime importance for this is the primary expression of 'suffering patient.' That is very marked in him, and perhaps that is what characterizes his case, although sometimes it may be a common symptom. The voice may communicate anxiety, restlessness and intensity of the suffering which should be noted. Again, a stress on a particular complaint, should be taken a note of. You have to prescribe for the voice. The voice holds the vital principle of the patient. In the conversation a repeated telling about a complaint on part of the patient should be marked and that symptom usually dominates the entire case, thus becoming uncommon.

The physician must inquire about certain important signs if the patient doesn't tell you, he should ask the patient or his relatives to inspect and describe. Tell him to palpate himself inspect himself or ask his relatives for help. Inquiry should also be made into his daily routine. And you may get some thread to your prescription. Interruptions should be avoided, they may disturb the chain of thought (as has also been advised by Master Hahnemann in the Organon of Medicine). The physician is expected to first listen what the patient says without interrupting him and after the patient has had his say he should go ahead with his questions. In no way the suffering patients dynamism and eagerness to tell his sufferings should be curbed because that's the only thing that will reveal everything behind the electronic veil. The patient who is in agony wants to express out his suffering and communicate everything to the physician and there lies the remedy in those one or two points he eagerly tells you. The 'flow' drives with itself the remedy to the physician.

Only when the picture of the patient's suffering doesn't get clear to the physician, the leading indications of specific remedies in the range that the physician has in mind may be asked. Certain leading questions may be asked in such cases if the patient misses on certain points.

The physician should ask the patient 'what was he doing just before he called the doctor and what would he like to do after it.' He may tell that he was getting his head pressed by somebody, or sleeping fully covered with a blanket or something like that giving you significant points about him. Or he may tell you that after his telephonic talk with the physician is over he may just want to lie down with closed windows and doors in complete dark and fully covered and you may have a remedy like Gelsemium ready for him to deliver cure.

The homeopath should write down the exact words of the patient. A read at the paper can instantly furnish him the right remedy. He should clarify the points that are not clear to him, and ask the patient if he has left anything.

One should never be in a hurry to prescribe a remedy immediately. You must tell the patient to call back after fifteen to twenty minutes in an acute case and a day or two in a chronic case. Broad-spectrum remedies should be thought of in such cases. The physician should try to speak in patient's language.

At the end of the conversation the patient should be asked to communicate if he wishes to tell anything. The patient should be instructed to call back if something has been left out and if he remembers something after a few minutes and wishes to convey it to the physician. In many cases that 'something,' may hold the remedy for him. There are certain things that the entire conversation conveys although the patient doesn't talk or refer to them. The physician must proceed with all the homeopathic inquiries that are necessary in acute cases and chronic cases.

Finally the physician must base his prescription on what he feels is important in the patient. It may be a combination of just a bitter mouth and thirstlessness calling for a remedy like Pulsatilla and bitter mouth and great thirst calling for Bryonia.

Prescribe on points that steal your maximum attention as a 'homeopathic' physician. 'Something', that stole the reason-gifted mind.

∎

CHAPTER 11

ONLINE PRESCRIBING

With everything under the sky available online homeopathic treatment is no exception. But a very little guiding information is available about it. Online prescribing can prove very beneficial and effective to manage long distance cases but more than anything, skill, perfection and extra care are necessary for it. It is the easiest and most convenient way of prescribing for long distance patients.

From acquiring the detailed history, to the selection of the remedy, every thing needs care and caution when prescribing for a patient whom you haven't actually seen.

Physicians should arrange at least the first visit of the patient and follow-up can be managed through web.

DESIGNING A WEBSITE

To design your own *web site* web page/site designers and other experts in the field should provide a dear help. Yet a physician needs to decide himself on how he wants his web site and has to guide the designers regarding how he wants the site.

On the Home page you may keep introductory articles/ paragraphs about homeopathic system of healing. Use of simple, easy, lucid and non-medical language. Attractive pictures in support of the articles should be added.

On the top user access options like *about us, contact us, sign up, treatment, about homeopathy, email* should be placed. It may also contain the basic information about your site. The main menu on the left hand side of the web page should include new advancements in medicine, health news, advancements in homeopathy, disease information, online questions. It is important to get the valid licence from the competent authority. There should always be a SEARCH option in your site, which should be very convenient for the user to delve into the site. At the bottom of the page your complete postal address along with email id should be there. The sight may be enriched with information about other exclusive websites related to homeopathic treatment and also reference books. A query section should make it more useful. Sentences from people about homeopathy can be displayed for example 'Homeopathy is the latest and most refined technique of treating patients economically and non violently"-M. K. Gandhi.

If you create your own website see to it that it is complete with the history form and instructions to the patient which should be preferably in multiple languages besides the English language, since internet users worldwide are likely to access the site. It should contain online form with a detailed questionare. Your website shouldn't carry too much of information which may confuse the patient who is new to the science, it should be relevant and to the point. It should cover the mode of treatment and may include certain articles about homeopathy as a science by yourself or by renowned people pioneers in the faculty. It should be replete with relevant facts. A physician may put an thoroughly received case may serve as a sample guideline for the patient.

The technology has its merits and demerits, pros and cons. This section takes a deep view of online prescribing.

ONLINE PRESCRIBING MERITS AND DEMERITS

MERITS

1. On line prescribing is a boon for long distance patients. People in rural places can consult expert urban physicians especially for their longstanding and obstinate ailments. Urban population can seek the treatment of experts in Metros just by sitting at home.

2. It is very convenient, time saving, energy saving and money saving too. Huge money spend on conveyance, travel lodging and boarding by long distance patients when they consult out of station physicians. It is a blessing for poor patients.

3. The patient has to refer the web site and this helps in spreading awareness about homeopathy, the disease awareness also increases.

4. You can consult a physician twenty-four hours and by your preference and time availability unlike direct consultation.

5. Through this type of consultation homeopathy and its benefits can spread to far off places and homeopathy can reach to millions of people.

6. When a patient is required to send/submit his history online he gets more thinking time and presents detailed history.

DEMERITS

1. A physician needs immense skill and intelligence to prescribe without actually seeing the patient. Errors in prescribing and diagnosis are more likely to occur.

2. Equipment failures and transmission glitches are likely to obstruct the treatment and produce unwanted interruptions.

3. Worldwide many regulations boards oppose ban internet prescribing for valid reasons hence it is difficult to get valid licence.

4. Many physicians find it time consuming difficult, and more complex than simple.

5. The technology is costly and many homeopathic doctors can't afford it. The set up and maintenance too is costly.

6. It is difficult to preserve confidentiality and personal information of the patient may be misused by hackers, or other internet mischief mongers and goons.

7. The 'Cybermedicine' prescribed by you may be misused and considered disease specific by the patient and used for himself or others injudiciously.

8. Designing web site using electronic system for prescribing is considered difficult inefficient than the direct prescribing / paper prescribing.

9. Physicians can advertise and make false and taller claims behind the webs.

10. Many world wide medical and pharmaceutical authorities caution patients from seeking foreign website prescribers and sites which prescribe medicines for the first time without examining the patient. They also warn not to provide personal information to such sites which may restrict them from using such online consultations.

How to overcome the Demerits

It is definitely not proper to prescribe a medicine without the physical examination of the patient even if his complete medical and homeopathic history is with you. So you can ask your patient to get himself thoroughly examined by a physician locally and enclose his report/ findings which can be greatly helpful to you.

The patient should be asked to send his complete medical reports. Scanned photographs and reports. An online prescription should only be made after a confirmed anamnesis and diagnosis by the physician. The case history of the patient can be recorded by video conferencing also, which has become very easy these days. A virtual chat or voice chat can be very helpful.

After a patient approaches you through Email first mail him the information necessary for homeopathic treatment, which should simply explain him in detail under all the heads that is necessary for homeopathic treatment. Tell him to send you a 'write up' of his complaints in an essay form liberally so that you have specific information. Then you can have specific questions. You can arrange a chat with him and get what can be called a 'chat history' there is nothing better than that. But here the patient gets every scope to hide certain details with some personal considerations especially the mental aspect his life space. Yet the chat history is very useful. You can store it in your floppy.

Getting the correct history is all that is important rest the case processing and selection of remedy remains the same. A physician may prescribe a remedy in a coded form.

MORE ON ONLINE PRESCRIBING

Government action against internet prescription is expected to be taken. Twenty seven out of seventy boards disciplined physicians for prescribing improperly since 1998. Hence 'Specific' or favourite remedies which have been found suitable in patients with specific diseases should not be administered through internet. Only the indicated remedy-simillimum should be administered in minimum doses.

According to Sure script systems include 6% of physicians prescribe electronically.

2 to 3% of 3 billion prescriptions are processed electronically.

HOMEOPATHY ON INTERNET

On the electronic globe too homeopathy has spread its dynamic world to a boundless degree. Homeopathy is available online in the form of following. One can get a very different vision about homeopathy through internet.

Homeopathic Web sites.

Articles E-books, online books.

Online directories.

Information about homeopathic software.

Online consultation web sites.

Websites of homeopathic institutions, associations and organizations in India and abroad.

Websites of online homeopathic education.

Homeopathy on internet can be explored by making a search "Homeopathy on Internet' or Homeopathic software Web sites' in suitable search engines like goggle. com, hotmail.com or rediff.com and hundreds of sites will be displayed which can be accessed with an easy click.

Following is a list of few useful homeopathic sites.

www.bjainbooks.com

(information about more than 5000 titles on homeopathy, health, alternative medicine and new age and business)

www.thespiritofhomeopathy.com/sankaran.html

www.abouthomeopathy.com/links.htm.

www.scientifichom.com/Links.htm

www.hpathy.com/LIBRARY/heopathy_library.asp

(for homeopathy books and e-books free download)

You can find best sites for homeopathic software through Starware Search which is a useful resource for finding. Again search can be made on Finindia.net.

■

CHAPTER 12

AIDS IN PRESCRIBING

We are into the age of computers, the age of electronic books, and specially designed software. The era of huge global network of knowledge. It will be very orthodox to think not to make a handy use these modern day aids. It won't be just correct and infact illogical to think that these computer programme don't give a scope to the physician to use his own mind and stall the use of his mental faculties, slowly making him dependent. In no way these homeopathic software programmes should be looked at with disdain. It won't be right to say that they simply serve the utility for the mediocre physicians crippled due deficient knowledge as well as intelligence.

In my view the use of every thing that helps the physician in the diagnosis and scientific selection of the remedy and thus ultimately benefits the patient should be encouraged. These aids often prove to be time saving and remove the troublesome mind blocks. The total dependence on these aids is something everyone is liable to and one should be careful about it. A physician may avail the useful help of these tools from time to time. These modern day tools not only help a homeopath to choose a remedy but they also widen the sphere of his knowledge. In every way they enhance the prescribing abilities of a physician and contribute greatly to development of his logical faculty.

They help in rapid repertorization. It's a direct, easy and convenient access to knowledge. These aids often come to respite in challenging situations. They also assist the physician to keep complete records – a detailed history and also the details of follow-ups. They also allow storing of relevant photographs of the patients and audio video records etc. Again the websites can also come to aid.

For the ultimate choice of the remedy a physician should employ his reason-gifted mind. The final selection of a remedy should be based on the physician's knowledge of materia medica, but the use of these aids should always be fruitful.

HANDY AIDS FOR PRESCRIBING

HOMPATH CLASSIC

This is a twenty one year old homeopathic software developed by Dr. Jawahar Shah of Bombay with 29 repertories, three hundred homeopathic books, five thousand articles and a one lakh plus pages of information. There is also a complete repertory by Roger Van Zandvoort.

It includes Archives, Homutil plus patient management system. One can also convert repertory into materia medica and vice versa. One can create his own repertory. It can also be used for a rapid global search within the full database. A case can be repertorized using same rubrics with different repertories to reach a sphere of remedies. Materia medica section can be helpful for final selection.

HOMPATH OZONE

This software contains Kent's repertory, Boericke's repertory, and has more than 2000 cross- references. Cost around Rs. 2795.00.

MATERIA MEDICA LIVE

This is a multimedia presentation CD with 21 remedies with a live presentation. The remedies have been divided into three groups Plant kingdom, Animal Kingdom and Mineral kingdom. Beautiful animation, effective sound and visual effects make it attractive and interactive.

CARA

This England based software is rich with Kent's repertory, Synthetic repertory, Boericke's Repertory, Phatak's Repertory, Boericke's Materia Medica, Phatak's MM, Kent's lectures and Allen's Key notes. It can greatly help a physician to analyze his case in multiple ways like by families of different salts like Kalis, Natrums, Ferrums, Calcareas etc. By classification snakes, plant, minerals, animals, nosodes etc. by periodic table Hydrogen series, Carbon series , Boron series, and even by miasms (Psora, sycotic syphilitic). It also includes some additional materia medicas. It also has Vithoulkas's additions to Kent's repertory.

CARALITE

It has a rare repertory known as combined repertory, which is based on Kent's repertory. The repertory has been expanded and additions made.

SIMILIA

This is useful to search and delve into different materia medica's.

RADAR

RADAR stands for Rapid Aid to Drug Aimed Research (RADAR). This homeopathic software includes VES Vithoulkas Expert System, rubrics can be analyzed through this system. It also has Materia Medica Viva, Synthesis Repertorium Homeopathicum Syntheticum Edited by Dr Frederik Schroyens. You can introduce changes in the database, you can register your symptoms in a repertorization and repertorize the case.

It has about 2000 remedies, some 260,000 additions, which have been derived from 320 different sources. EXILIBRIS - reaching for the stars, this includes all the books available in English.

POLYCHRESTA

It has been developed by Thane base Cybernetic systems pvt. limited and contains 5 repertories, 6 Materia Medica's and lots of useful information.

ORGANON 96

This programme has been developed by Dr. Dilip Dixit of Institute of clinical research Bombay and based on ICR's Standardized Case Record (SCR) system.

A homeopath should use his discretion to select any of the above programme for his use depending on his need for help. He should assess the individual utility of the programmes and select one for him. All the above software programmes are handy, complete, and useful in many ways.

CHAPTER 13

A GOOD DOCTOR, A GOOD PRESCRIBER

> This section deals with an entirely new aspect of healing, which must be looked into by professional healers of all faculties of medicine. In the rapidly changing times things are becoming grossly commercial, people are losing faith in the professional healers. And today perhaps people are looking for a good doctor first than an expert physician so it is becoming increasingly important that a physician should be 'a good doctor' first. It is the time when we need to put in untiring perseverance to bring back this faith in us, which is being lost.

Some years back even if you had a trivial health problem in no time you could call a doctor at your home. You could get his medical advice and not just that but you would also be getting free doses of sympathy, friendly boosts and a warm touch of concern without paying him any extra fee. You could even share some good time with him over a cup of tea. With such 'treatment' one could be much better even before taking the prescribed treatment of the doctor.

Today it's a totally different scenario. For patients things have changed a lot. They need to take a prior appointment of the 'Busy' doctor (which implies you need to fall ill as per doctor's availability and schedule). They get to see his face only after a long wait, after they have swallowed the entire stuff of the glossy magazines in his waiting room. What follows next is not very encouraging. The doctor advises him some investigations X-rays, USGs and some pathological tests and asks you to come back with their reports. So another appointment, another wait.

He goes back to him with his reports and doctor gives him hardly ten minutes out of his busy clock only to tell him that you are suffering from common cold and no other big disease. He prescribes some drugs (by this time he may be much better). After much efforts and waiting he receives the treatment from a medical professional but hardly gets the 'doctors advice', his care, his time which he really wants.

This may seem to be an exaggeration but the situation today is no different. When an ill, distressed, suffering person comes to a doctor what he really needs at such time is not just the correct prescription as is the case with many a homeopaths today, neither he wants a shopping list of drugs prescribed. It is really not the only thing for which he wants a doctor's consultation.

Hence a good prescriber should also be a good doctor first otherwise even after making a correct prescription for his patient, the patient may not totally recover from his ailment. It is important that along with the dynamic remedy administered by him his dynamic force, 'will' is able to contribute to the healing through his heartfelt words, nice behaviour and sincere advice. In a science, that believes on existence of a dynamic force in human beings, and medicine this is very important for a cure. A doctor needs to put his spiritual energies in the patient. Motivate him positively towards the cure. He needs to make a good use of his will power. And it hold great significance in this spiritual science.

What a patient really needs is a good 'treatment' a kind, comforting, consolatory advice. What he needs from the doctor is care, consideration and concern for his ailment. Besides the medical treatment he needs another treatment, which should include high power drugs of sympathy and empathy and health tonics like, positive assurance and boosting words. A patient who is in agony, in an intense suffering needs a doctor's friendly touch, he needs some comforting words from doctor, which can be magical. What he needs is a motivation to get well soon and recommence his healthy life. Sadly a patient going to a doctor doesn't get any of these things.

All these can really prove to be wonder drugs. These drugs, which were invented far before Hippocrates invented life-giving drugs, can act miraculously. Hence if one really wishes to be an expert prescriber, he must also try to gain expertise in this very art. They can influence the process of cure in their own way. Unfortunately very few doctors are consciously making their use today. The physician has to satisfy his susceptibility for all the above needs.

In the past doctors were appreciated and recognized for a good sense of humour. They could be even making a patient in intense agony laugh at his own suffering. Only a few doctors use good humour today. A clinician should make his patient laugh with a talk that has an iota of humour. Today most of physicians assume a stiff posture, a sort of serious formal attitude. This further widens the distance between the two ends of the doctor's table to a boundless extent. A doctor while dealing with a patient needs to be a human being first and then a doctor. He needs to be most natural and friendly while dealing with his patient. Only a human touch and not a professional one can bring a doctor closer to a patient, which is very essential for making a doctor understand patient's malady in depth. This is also important as regards to the securing of the personal information from the patient, which is relevant in making a correct prescription.

A good communication and the establishment of a comfort zone between the doctor and the patient are very essential. Many a times there is a communication gap between a doctor and the patient which if much widened can prove to be an obstacle in treatment. A bottom heart welcome smile from a doctor can make a patient forget his suffering for a time. A put on the back can do wonders to his confidence.

A doctor needs to be transparent while dealing with his patients. He should be explaining the patient in detail about his disease though he may skip some part for the benefit of the patient for good reasons. He should also inform him about the nature of the treatment, and also make him aware about the principles of the science. He should explain in detail the nature of the cure he is going to offer to him. He should tell him why certain phenomenon are happening and are likely to happen and why the patient need not worry about them.

He should be relieving the patient of all his anxieties about his disease. He should provide him ample hope, which is scarcely visible to him in the dusk of despair. The image of the doctor in mind of the patient should be the one of a dear uncle, a good friend, a kind sympathizer and not just a medicinal professional. He should explain to the patient how the remedy administered by him will act, he should be transparent with him only then can a relationship of trust be established between him and the patient.

It is very important that a physician instills confidence in his patient and makes him feel that he can relieve his suffering effectively. Unfortunately with the mushrooming grow of health institutes and diagnostic centers patients are missing all this. Health care is loosing the care part. The family doctor concept is slowing being dumped into back seats with doctors finding a little time to attend their patients. A physician besides being courageous and principled should always keep in mind that he is dealing with dynamism- remedies that have a dynamic action on the patient's dynamic vital force. He should divert all his dynamic positive energies towards healing. He should instill confidence and sketch a promising picture in front of the patient thereby make his thoughts positive. Make him feel that his disease is trivial as far a treating and getting well is concerned.

A patient should be clearly able to see 'a confidence in his physician' which has its own significance in curing. The physician's immense faith in the science and confidence in himself should be reflected in his demeanor only than can he expect his patient to be a believer in the science and the doctor professing it. Medical treatment today lacks this human touch. A human touch more than just medical advice can do wonders in the science of healing. It may not be life saving but can certainly enliven the patient. Give him life in this way.

BEING 'THE COURAGEOUS DOCTOR'

Anxieties often distress and disturb the physician often leading to vexation, agitation and lowering the performance, capabilities and competence of the physician. A physician should try to consciously eradicate them from his mind. A physician should always imagine a cure and not failure waiting ahead for him. He should remember that anxieties are natural for every physician.

He should try to remain cool. Take deep long breaths. Drink plenty of water. Only positive and intellectual thinking can help them to whip away the anxieties.. With experience, and expertise these anxieties are slowly described.

Only the faith in the science and its principles and in his scientific selection can make one shrug of fear of all kinds.

Constantly re-assuring self that 'Nothing shall happen,' when your patient is under your treatment and if the accepted case is well within the domain of homeopathy, can be very comforting.

Previous good performance and successful treatments should be remembered. A physician should never carry the anxieties home and lastly, to the bed. He should be able to 'shut off' no sooner he reaches home.' However, reasonable anxieties often help the physician and drive him to make extra efforts and thinking in the process benefiting cure. They also guide him to be a little more cautious.

Knowledge is the only weapon against all kinds of fears and anxieties lest a physician is a weak individual. Only a knowledgeable physician can be a bold and courageous physician, a 'Man of Steel.' You can win over the disease only if you believe you can. So believe in your self and remember only a calm mind can be an intelligent one.

■

CHAPTER 14

WHAT YOUNG MEN CAN OFFER TO HOMEOPATHY ?

A YOUNG MAN'S ANSWER TO DR. ROBERTS' QUESTION

Dr. Herbert Roberts in the very first chapter of his masterpiece "The Principles and Art of Cure by Homeopathy," asks 'What homeopathy has to offer the young man ?' He says if the young man wants to use his foothold as a physician for a life of ease for fame and riches homeopathy has to offer him nothing. But he says that to the young man who is equipped and wiling to undergo these training which includes hours of study of philosophy and patient study, tracing the course of the disturbance and the remedy to fit in it for his lifelong task, homeopathy has everything to offer. It offers a life of service to humanity. It offers the independent mind an opportunity continually to seek new verifications of the natural laws upon which, this system of medicine is based. What homeopathy has to offer to you depends upon what you have to offer to homeopathy.

He mentions that Homeopathy as a profession carries a challenge. The possibilities of art are infinite. He concludes the chapter on a questioning note- *Young man, what have you to offer homeopathy?*

'**Everything**' is a one word answer, I think my young heart ejects out. Yes a young man can offer everything to homeopathy provided he realizes that it is a privilege, a rare opportunity and honour to be a homeopath. A young man should understand that it is not by chance he has come in the faculty, he is destined for it. It is with a pure purpose that he has been chosen to be a homeopath. All young men must consider homeopathy as a blessing, an opportunity of lifetime to do something.

But the basic question is does homeopathy as a science really need anything from us? Is it incomplete or isn't it complete in all aspects. Homeopathy as a science is surely complete in all respects and nothing extra can be added to it. Fundamentally what we can offer to homeopathy is the application of the principles of this great science, which are unfortunately being forgotten and dumped in the back seats by the physician of the faculty. This is what young man can basically offer to homeopathy.

I think primarily we all owe three responsibilities towards the science:

1. Preserving its philosophical integrity,
2. promoting its scientific development, and
3. spreading its popularity.

It is for the young physician of today to realize these three responsibilities and try to shoulder them. It will be a great offering of the young man to homeopathy.

It is sad to note that presently there is a sorry state of affairs in homeopathy. There are multiple methods of practice, innumerable confusions, unskilled physician are misguiding their students, unscientific prescribing, untrained teachers and ill equipped institutions exist. Many misconceptions have stuck hard in the minds of the people, many believe that severe aggravation of complaints is a must in homeopathic treatment, many feel homeopathy 'takes out' all the diseases of the body through skin (thanks to the favourite remedies of the senior practitioners). Perhaps we are nearing a day when the misconceptions about the science shall rise so high that disbelief will emerge. We may loose the science one day. This is something the young men have to prevent.

But it is really pleasing to see that today's young homeopaths are not ready to accept the 'split second prescriptions' delivered at the clinics of the so called experienced and famous homeopaths. These crowd pulling physicians who have a long lane of patients infront of their clinics (like a cinema hall) hardly seem to satisfy the intelligent budding homeopaths with their ways of practice.

Gone are the days when young physicians used to get satisfied when their 'practitioner gurus' had one answer to every prescription. 'Today's young homeopath have a desire to seek the truth and I feel this is a greatest natural gift to homeopathy from the young doctors. This intense desire is worth praising and it can lead to great heights.

Today's young homeopath is courageous enough to ask straightaway his seniors who don't practice what they preach in their theory-why don't they practice as per the guidelines of Dr. Hahnemann.

Unfortunately many experienced senior physicians have no clear-cut specific answers to the very simple, straightforward genuine questions asked by the budding homeopaths. What is their experience of any use when they cannot logically justify and give a reason why they have prescribed a particular remedy. What kind of experience they are talking of? Dr. Kent says 'Unless man has truth in his mind his experiences are false. Truth in the mind is first and then experiences are good. You cannot trust the experience of men who do not know what is true neither can they be led into truth by theses fallacious experiences.

Many of popular homeopaths in spite of having great rush at their clinics have not been able to establish a graceful position for homeopathy. Well how can they by prescribing Calc. for obesity and Bar-c. for dwarfism. They have little to offer to their patients and homeopathy. I am sad that homeopathy is being brutally murdered at such clinics, which are famous as '*Mecca* of homeopathy', which offer a cure for everything under the sky.

Homeopathy is on the death bed and only young blood can revive it. Many of these clinics, which are able to generate rush though aggressive marketing, giving false hope to patients and making tall claims are doing no good to homeopathy. Many patients come here with a hope and leave, in disappointment and unfortunately many feel that they can never be cured by homeopathy because they have tried the best option. They feel there is no better homeopathy beyond that. It is the responsibility of young minds to erase these wrong impressions of the patients with their right approach, and right guidance.

Of late, there has been a marked change in the map of Homeopathy in India, it is no more the country where those popular homeopaths, the routinists who prescribe their favourite one, two or even three remedies in minutes, something with which neither they nor their patient is satisfied.

Slowly but surely it is also emerging into a country where young homeopaths are practicing homeopathy scientifically as per the guidelines of Organon. Today's homeopaths record the detailed history of their patients, they thoroughly examine their patients, they advise investigation wherever needed, they correctly arrive at a diagnosis, they go ahead with making a totality and repertorization of a case. These young homeopathic healers are able to leave a very good impression on their patients because they can advise them rightly, because they don't make tall claims, and don't misguide their patients with false promises.. This is the sort of homeopathy young men can offer to people. This scientific homeopathy will be a greatest tribute to Dr Hahnemann from the young.

Since I was a child I have been hearing it from people, 'homeopathy is developing' in spite of it being a 'developed science.' Decades have past and I am still hearing 'homeopathy is developing.' By this time what we should really hear about a science, that is already a developed one, is that 'homeopathy has really developed.' This proves that in all these long years the incompetent physicians have not been able to deliver in full and have stalled the development of the science. A young man has this responsibility to replace the primary health care with a developed homeopathy. I feel it is now very much a responsibility of young shoulders to see that homeopathy is a developed science in the eyes of the people. A young man has this responsibility to replace the primary health care with a developed homeopathy. It can be a great offering.

Every young man has some personal wealth he can offer to homeopathy. By personal wealth I mean those rare attributes, the qualities, which only you as a person have. A young man has himself to offer to homeopathy, his sky scraping spirits as a youth, his entire life. He can offer his new vision, his qualities of youth the determination, the inquisitiveness, the logical mind, the insight, the industriousness, the boldness to accept challenges, his inherent talents, his dedication, devotion, his positive attitude, energetic efforts and exceptional enthusiasm, his imagination and what not. It is the need of the science.

Dr. Roberts has said in his very first chapter that one of the outstanding problems is cancer. This is a challenge to homeopathic physician. He has this field of work, which offers much elbowroom. And going by what he has suggested, the young spirited enthusiastic young homeopaths can go ahead with their research on treatment of cancer with homeopathy. They can explore this in greater depths.

The trio of hard work, intelligence and honesty can well serve the cause of homeopathy. And a young man can offer them whole heartedly to homeopathy. With a right approach a young man can become not only a famous homeopath in a city but also around the globe. Today homeopathy needs more young scientists than the old artists. Homeopathy needs real research under right guidance. Not the one displayed on the boards of some clinics and institutions these days.

Homeopaths today must reflect a scientific touch, a magnificent expression of their knowledge through their methodical approach, through their decent behaviour and elegant presentation in front of the patient. Homeopathy is a speciality and we need to pose and dress like specialists.

What young man can offer to homeopathy is the right method of practice as per the Organon of medicine. Every homeopath must ask a question to himself 'Whether he is rightly doing his practice' and the answer will guide him to what he can really offer to homeopathy. They need to maintain proper and complete records and this way can do great research work. They must carry on with continuing medical education, apply principles of homeopathy in newer emerging diseases, gather real knowledge by organizing seminars, conferences, interactions, clinical meeting, case discussions. They must promote that homeopathy is simple and not complicated and complex as is the general opinion. Guide the directionless juniors and ignorant seniors. What a young man can do is spread the light of right homeopathy, the homeopathy practiced according to the guidelines of the Dr. Hahnemann not only amongst people but also among the fellow practitioners of other faculty who look down upon homeopathy with disdain. Young men must increase self-belief and faith of other people in the science. They can make the science richer by their efforts.

They can accept challenges from the sick and suffering sections of medicine, explore newer areas, like learning how to record a history where the patient is deaf and dumb or imbecile. Devise a method to investigate mentals of patient from rural and lower socio-economic strata. Young homeopaths must use the modern day developments in science and technology for better application of the science. They must use the research in other fields for betterment of homeopathy. Homeopathy is our beloved and respected mother we need to practice it as a science, and not disrespect it by just considering it an art and prescribe as per our wishes.

The first thing they should do is to search for themselves a proper guide who is not a hypocrite and really practices what he preaches. They should look for institutions, which provide standardized training. They can unmask the faces of the hippocrates and quacks in the faculty so that good stands and prospers, and the bad is exposed and eradicated and the science of homeopathy is saved. Only a scientific homeopathy has the potentials to mobilize the masses towards the science, only good brings good, as is a universal law.

A young man has to offer himself to homeopathy as skilled physician and honest person. As Dr. Roberts says if he has heart to serve humanity with sincerity of purpose irrespective of returns I am sure he may find fame and riches at his door as well also a place of honour a well-earned place in the community. Homeopathy will also reward him handsomely.

The proper understanding and application of homeopathic philosophy by young men can make us see the light of the day when principled, scientific, honest and unprejudiced physicians will be healing the humanity with Hahnemannian cure.

PRACTICAL DEMONSTRATION OF A THOROUGHLY WORKED CASE

DETAILS OF THE PATIENT

Name: Mrs. Disha Deshpande (name changed)

Age: 32 years, Married (1986) Female.

Hindu, Non vegetarian.

Spouse: Mr. Deshpande. Age: 43 years, Occupation: Chemist.

Father: 59 years, Teacher, was in seoni.

Mother: 54 years, Housewife.

B_1 21 year S_2 34 years, both married .

Children: M 5 years, F 13 years.

CHIEF COMPLAINT

At 28 years age

After 2nd Pregnancy	Pain[3+] throbbing	< Sun[2+]
Head	Heaviness and	< Afternoon[2+] Night[3+]

	burning	(during rest)
	Giddiness[2+]	< Anger[2+] and vexation[2+]
		< On fast days[2+]
Sensorium		> When mentally occupied
Vertex		> when working[2+]
(shifting)		> After sleep
		> closing windows and doors darkness[2+]

CONCOMITANT

Sleep loss of, twitching and weakness of limbs, fear something will happen to her, fear of becoming crazy.

ASSOCIATED COMPLIANTS

		< Winter[3+]
Since school days	Vesicular eruptions, Itching	< Soap
Legs, hands, skin	Cracks, rough skin	< Warm water dipping in
	burning and occa-sional bleeding	< Touch of Brinjals cooking while
		> Rainy season.

PATIENT AS A PERSON

General appearance
Thin build, fair complexion
Ht. 5'4", WT. 45 Kg

Appetite and Thirst
Normal

Craving
Salty^{3+} and spicy^{3+} food
Fish^{2+}, Milk

Aversion
Sweets except milk (Khoya based) sweets.

Addiction
tea 4 to 5 cups a day since her younger days.

ELIMINATIONS

Stools
Soft but not satisfactory, formed sticky sometimes foamy, losses stools with gurgling in abdomen, pain in abdomen before stools.

Urine
Occasional burning < summer Odour $^{2+}$

Sweats
On face axilla no odor, no stains.

MENSTRUAL FUNCTION
Menarche 9th stand
LMP 30/8/2000

Complaints
BM Tenderness breast.
DM Pain in back and extremities and exhaustion.
Cycles 18-28 days.
5-6 days duration.
Flow scanty, red stain brownish difficult to wash, clots dark red no odor.

F - 10

H/O Excessive discharge / white mucoid < after first delivery. She has been cauterized thrice in 6-7 years for this complaint < After menses.

Pregnancy

Both normal, frequent bleeding during pregnancy was advised rest.

Lochia^{2+}, breast fed till 1½ years.

Sexual function

Two or three days a week, satisfaction$^+$, no complains during and after.

Sleep and dreams

Not always sound and refreshing often disturbed because of fear of thieves. Husband is out of town wakes with fright but not because of dreams.

Dreams not remembered.

Physical reactions

< Drafts^{2+}

< sun = Headache^2

Bathing-warm bath all through the year except sever summers. Moderate warm drinks, averse to cold drinks and ice cream prefers moderate temperature.

Likes rains but not storms, and humid weather.

PAST HISTORY

Nothing peculiar.

FAMILY HISTORY

F 59 Koch's disease.

M54 Flatulence, acidity Chronic backache piles.

S_1S_2 Susceptible to colds.

S_2 HBP, Obesity.

B Eosinophilia.

The patient didn't know about the details of other except the very near relatives.

PHYSICAL FINDINGS

Pulse: 70/min.

B.P.: 110/70 mm of Hg.

Tongue: Slight yellow coating posteriorly.

Throat: Slight enlarged tonsils.

Nails: Longitudinal ribbed.

Skins of palms lesion red small eruptions, yellow brown spots, dry wrinkled skin cracks.

LIFE SPACE

All the points of LS have been included in Mental interpretations.

CASE ANALYSIS, EVALUATION AND INTERPRETATIONS

DIAGNOSIS

I. Vascular headache without aura

Factors in favour of diagnosis

1. Attacks of severe headache with throbbing pain[3+].
2. Headache aggravated by sun[3+] and fasting days[2+].
3. Headache ameliorated by sleep and closing windows and doors.

II. Chronic Irritant contact dermatitis

Factors in favour of diagnosis

1. Red, vesicular eruptions on legs and hands since childhood.
2. Cracked and rough skin.
3. Itching.
4. Aggravation from contact of soap and brinjals.

THERMALS

Patient's expression	Hot	Ambithermal	Chilly
Bathing-takes warm bath all through			
The years excepts severe summer			*
Prefers warm bath			
Covers varies with season but desires light			*
Covers throughout the year till chest			
Averse to chilled drinks, Ice cream.			
Takes moderately warm drinks			*
Prefers moderate temperature		*	
< Drafts^2			*
< Sun^2= CC	*		

INTERPRETATION OF MIND

Phase	Situation	Reaction	Interpretation
C H I L D H O O D	At school	She was afraid of teachers and because of it regularly did homework.	Fear
		She had many friends, participated in sports.	Social
	At Home	She was not in the habit of working, was lazy and averse to work.	Indolent
	Performance in Studies	She passed HSC in second division completed B.Com In first attempt.	Mediocre
	Aspirations	She wanted to become a doctor, do job wants to improve her confidence and be like other women.	Ambitious
A D U L D H O O D	Employment	She did teachership after marriage. Worked as an accountant in a private firm.	Normal response
		Lost interest in doing job after children were born.	Normal response
	When she is working	She is anxious and tense whether she will do the work properly.	Anxiety
	When guests are expected	She is very tense before their arrival and thinks whether she will be able to meet their demands.	Anticipatory Anxiety

Patients version about herself	She is afraid to go out alone and gets. Palpitation if nervous.	Anxiety Timid
	She has no confidence in herself.	Lack of confidence
Thunderstorms and Lightening.	She fears them.	Fear of thunderstorms and lightening.
When Children disobey or contradict her if things don't go the way she wants.	She gets angry She feels disheartened and thinks she has no importance in house.	Anger Discouraged
Regarding her efforts.	She is conscious that she is at error yet she don't have the humility to accept and become adamant.	Unreasonable Fear and Anxiety.
If scolded by Husband in presence of others.	She feels terribly insulted and caries the vexation for days.	Agitated
Trivial matters	She gets rebuked over trivial matters that can be over looked she gets angry and argues.	Sensitive
Regarding problems	She is not able to erase them from memory and keeps recalling them even after they are solved she is never satisfied with the outcome of problems.	Brooding Vexation Dissatisfaction

When she is angry regarding the work about her sister.	She goes out of control wants to beat, strike children.	Excitable
	She is lazy in work and hates to do any kind of work.	Indolent
	She is envious of her as she looks after her father in law all and always gets praises.	Envious
She feels that	She is worthless and is unable to contribute in any manner in the house.	Depression
Her efforts to improve herself	She thinks of doing many things for it but her enthusiasm dampened even before she begins. Doesn't feel like doing any work.	Lacks Motivation
When using electrical equipments	She fears she may get a shock.	Fear

Conclusion;- Patient Ambithermal towards chilly [4+].

The following mental state and mental evolution was drawn from the above expression

MENTAL STATE

Intellect: Mediocre

Ambitious

Emotions: Anxiety, Fear

Behaviour: Social

Functioning: Indolent

MENTAL EVOLUTION

Lack of motivation

Poor performance

Dissatisfaction

Agitation

Excitable

Anger

Vexation

Sensitive

Unreasonable

Envy

Fear: Of thunderstorms and lightening

Of thieves

That something will happen to her

Of death

Of becoming crazy

Anticipatory anxiety

Discouraged

Lack of confidence

Brooding

Depression

Generalization

The following modalities having sufficient intensity have been considered from the patient chief complaint and associated complaints and generalized in the given case.

$< $ Suppressed anger^{2+}

$<$ At rest^{2+}

$<$ Sun^{2+}

$<$ Winter^{2+}

$<$ Drafts^{2+}

$>$ When mentally occupied^{2+}

TOTALITY OF SYMPTOMS

FAMILY HISTORY

F- Koch's disease M- Piles, Acidity, chronic backache S_1 and S_2 Susceptible to colds

B_1 Hypertension, Obesity

B_2 Eosinophilia

PAST HISTORY

Frequent bleeding during second pregnancy

Excessive bleeding for 25- days, 1 year back dilatation and curettage done.

Cauterization done thrice in last 6-7 years for excessive leucorrhoea which $<$ after first delivery.

Eczema since childhood.

MENTAL STATE

Intellect: Mediocre

              Ambitious

Emotions: Anxiety, Fear

Behaviour: Social

Functioning: Indolent

THERMALITY

Ambithermal towards chilly.

1. GENERALS

MODALITIES

Aggravation

< Suppressed anger^{2+}

< At rest^{2+}

< Sun^{2+}

< Winter^{2+}

< Drafts^{2+}

Amelioration

> When mentally occupied^{2+}

MENTAL EVOLUTION

Lack of motivation

Poor performance

Dissatisfaction

Agitation

Excitable

Anger

Vexation

Sensitive

Unreasonable

Envy

Fear: Of thunderstorms and lightening

Of thieves

That something will happen to her

Of death

Of becoming crazy

Anticipatory anxiety

Discouraged

Lack of confidence·

Brooding

Depression

PHYSICAL

Craving for Fish^{2+}

Aversion sweets chilled drinks and ice cream.

Addiction to tea^{2+} since she was young.

Sleep not refreshing.

Disturbed because of fear of thieves, wakes up with fright when alone.

2. CHARACTERISTIC PARTICULARS

A. MODALITIES

Aggravation

< Suppressed anger^{2+}

< vexation

< At rest^{2+}

< Sun^{2+}

< Winter^{2+}

< Drafts^{2+}

Amelioration

> When mentally occupied[2+]

SENSATION

Headache[2] throbbing, shifting pain.

Giddiness[2.]

Heaviness of head and burning.

CONCOMITANTS

Mentals

Fear something will happen to her.

Fear of death and of becoming crazy.

Physical

Twitching of limbs.

Sensation as if limbs have no strength.

Trembling of body.

Location

Head, Sensorium.

B. MODALITIES

< Winter[2+]

< Exposure to warm water.

< Evening after rising from bed.

Rainy season.

Sensation

Red vesicular eruptions, skin dry rough and cracked.

Yellow, brown spots.

Itching burning on scratching occasional bleeding.

Location

Skin, Extremities .

C. TONSILS ENLARGED

D. MODALITY

< Before stools.

Sensation

Pain in abdomen.

Unsatisfactory stools.

Location

Bowels.

E. URINE OFFENSIVE, FREQUENT URGE

Burning during urination.

Location

Urinary system

F. MODALITY

< After Menses.

Sensation

Menses - Scanty, red coloured discharge brownish stains difficult to wash.

Dark coloured spots.

Leucorrhoea profuse, white mucoid.

Concomitants

Pain in back and extremities.

Tenderness of breasts before menses.

Location

Female Genital organs.

G. NAILS RIBBED LONGITUDINALLY

Selection of Repertory.

In the given case the following qualified mentals were found.

< Suppressed anger^{2+} – an emotional aggravating modality.

< Vexation – an emotional aggravating modality.

> When mentally occupied^{2+} a mental ameliorating modality.

Fear something will happen to her.

Fear of death and of becoming crazy mental concomitants in a physical complaint hence important.

Hence Kent's repertory has been selected for repertorization.

For potential differential field Kent's repertory has been used as it cover the symptoms considered in PDF.

REPERTORIAL TOTALITY- KENT'S REPERTORY

No.	Symptom	Rubric	Chapter	P. no
1	< Suppressed anger	ailments after, anger, Vexation etc.	MIND	2
2	< Sun^{2+}	Sun, from exposure to	GENERALITIES	1404
3	< Drafts^{2+}	Air, Draft agg	GENERALITIES	1344
4	< At rest^{2+}	Rest	GENERALITIES	1397
5	> When Mentaily occupied^{2+}	Occupation, amel	MIND	69
6	Fear of death	Fear, death of	MIND	44
7	Fear of becoming crazy	Fear, insanity of	MIND	45

Potential Differential Field – Kent's Repertory

No.	Symptom	Rubric	Chapter	Page no
1	Craving for fish	Desires fish	STOMACH	485
2	Nails ribbed longitudinally	Corrugated nails	EXTREMITIES	970
3	Addiction tea[2+]	Desires tea	STOMACH	486
4	Leucorrhoea profuse < after menses[2]	Leucorrhoea, menses after	GENITALIA FEMALE	722
5	Fear of thunderstorms	FEAR, thunderstorms of	MIND	47
6	Fear of thieves	Fear, Robbers of	MIND	47
7	Tenderness of breasts before menses	Pain, mammae, menses before	CHEST	846

After the repertorization the remedies scoring more than 1/3 rd of the highest marks covered were differentiated into acute and chronic and further into chilly hot and ambithermal remedies the patient being chilly the chronic chilly and ambithermal remedies were considered for PDF.

Following are the chronic chilly remedies that have prominently emerge in PDF:

1. Conium-7/3
2. Calcarea carb-6/2
3. Silicea – 6/3
4. Phosphorus – 8/3

COMPARISON OF CALCAREA CARB WITH THE PATIENT

COMPARISON AT MENTAL LEVEL

If we compare the patient's mind with Calcarea mind we find that our patient is intellectually mediocre and an ambitious person. In Calc. we find a dull intellect but like our patient a Calc. individual is also ambitious. Anxiety and fear, which are basic emotions in our patient are marked in Calc.. In our patient we find that an indolent functioning the patient being very slow in her work and doesn't like to work. In Calc. we find a basic slowness and inability to apply oneself on time. The patient is not desirous to work and lands in failure, similar is the case in our patient in whom her indolent functioning coupled with lack of motivation has lead to a poor performance. If we consider the expressions of our patient we find that the marked expressions are dissatisfaction excitability, anger, vexation, envy, fear of becoming crazy, fear of death, anticipatory anxiety, discouragement, brooding, depression. In Calc. fear of becoming crazy and fear of death are marked.

In our patient we find that owing to a poor performance that our patient is dissatisfied and agitated and has become excitable, she is angry and vexed, she has become a sensitive person. This has given rise to the feeling of envy, the patient is at times unreasonable. Fear, anxiety and lack of confidence is the final outcome of all this.

If we closely observe Calc. mind we find that in Calc. irritability vexation and frustration arise after failure. Owing to his failure the patient develops feelings of insecurity, anxiety and fear. Unable to succeed himself, he harbour's feelings of hostility, envy, jealousy and suspicion about the people who succeed.

Our patient is envious of her elder sister who takes good care of her FIL while she herself cannot do so. Calc. patient is unable to achieve what he desires resorts to corrupt practices, all this finally bring sadness, dejection and guilt and he becomes indifferent and apathetic avoids society and sits brooding. In our patient we find that depression and lack of confidence is the resultant of all the emotional disturbance, she too as Calc. keeps brooding but unlike calc our patient hasn't become totally indifferent and mixes with neighbours though she has not remained as social as she was previously.

COMPARISON OF PHYSICAL GENERALS

Calc is a chilly remedy while the patient is ambithermal towards chilly. Amongst modalities of the patient that have been generalized < suppressed anger^{2+} < sun^{2+} < while rest $^{2+}$ > mental occupation^{2+} < draft are covered by Calc. < draft being marked in Calc. Though Calc. covers > mental occupation and < mental exertion is marked in Calc. in whom exertion in general aggravates. Amongst the cravings and aversions of the patient none can be found in Calc. Craving for eggs and indigestible things and aversion to meat is characteristic of calc. The General unrefreshing sleep and disturbed sleep waking frequently with fright are covered by Calc. waking up with fright is prominent in Calc.

COMPARISON OF CHARACTERISTIC PARTICULARS

Considering the particulars of the patient Calc. has prominent action on head and sensorium, throbbing headache with vertigo is prominent in Calc. Calc. covers shifting pain with giddiness. The sensation burning in vertex is characteristic of Calc.

The concomitants trembling and twitching of limbs with weakness are prominent sensations in Calc. Amongst the sensations of skin Calc. covers vesicular eruption with itching burning and occasional Bleeding, dry rough and chapped skin is characteristic of Calc. Amongst the particular modalities< winter is marked in Calc. Calc. lacks > rainy season. In our patient we find < evening

F - 11

after rising from bed in Calc. < morning on waking is marked. Calc lacks < warm water dipping in.

Considering the other particulars enlargement of tonsils is a marked sensation in Calc. The sensation unsatisfactory stools with pain in abdomen before stools is covered by Calc. and also well marked in Calcarea. Calcarea covers the particular burning in urination with frequent urge and offensive urine, offensive urine is prominent in Calc. The particular leucorrhoea white profuse< after menses^{2+} is marked in Calc. Amongst the menstrual complaints of the patient, Calc covers scanty menses but profuse early menses is marked in Calc. In Calc. ailments from suppressed menses is prominent. Amongst the concomitants Calc. cover pain in back and extremities during menses. The concomitant tenderness of breasts before menses is characteristic in Calc. the peculiar sensation ribbed nails is lacking in calc.

Calcarea is preeminently a sycotic medicine and has also tubercular and psoric expressions.

After comparison of the remedies it is found that Calc carb. resemble the patient most. But it differs with thermality hence Calcarea sulph. which is an ambithermal remedy of Calcarea group was compared but it did not resemble the patient hence giving a consideration to the miasmatic background Calcarea phos. was also compared with the patient. Further a closer look was taken into the physical reactions of the patient and it was found that < sun^{2+} and preferring moderate temperature are the two hot and ambithermal reactions while rest are chilly < sun is well covered by Calcarea.

Calcarea resembles the patient. It is the overall picture of the patient that resembles one cannot get the exact or closest similarity.

ACUTE TOTALITY

a) Modalities:

    Aggravation: < Suppressed anger[2+]

                    < vexation

                    < At rest[2+]

                    < Sun[2+]

                    < Winter[2+]

                    < Drafts[2+]

    Amelioration: > When mentally occupied[2+].

    Sensation:

Headache[2+] throbbing, shifting pain.

Giddiness[2+].

Heaviness of head and burning.

Concomitants:

    Mentals: Fear something will happen to her.

                Fear of death and of becoming crazy.

    Physical: Twitching of limbs.

                Sensation as if limbs have no strength.

                Trembling of body.

    Location: Head, Sensorium.

Following acute chilly remedies were compared with the patient

    Belladonna

    Gelsemium

    Ignatia

    Nux vomica

    Rhus tox

COMPARISON OF THE SELECTED REMEDY

If we compare Ignatia with the patient we find that it has prominent action on head. Headache is a prominent sensation in Ignatia. Ignatia covers patient sensations giddiness. Amongst the other sensations Ignatia coves throbbing and shifting pain . Heaviness of head and burning in head sensation as if a nail was driven out through side of the head is characteristic of Ignatia. Amongst the modalities of the patient Ignatia covers < suppressed anger^{2+}, Vexation < Sun^{2+} < Drafts^{2+}, <while at rest and amel. when mentally occupied. Aggravation from suppressed anger and vexation are marked in Ignatia . Amongst the concomitants Ignatia covers fear of death and fear of becoming crazy. The concomitant twitching of limb, trembling and weakness areas is characteristic in Ignatia.

RELATIONSHIP OF IGNATIA WITH CALCAREA CARB.

Ignatia is related to Calcarea carb.$^{3+}$ (Reference B Therapeutic pocket Book).

Following detailed case has been give work out the case and select the remedy.

CASE FOR WORKING

Study, analyze, evaluate the following case, prepare totality, repertorial totality and PDF compare the emerging remedies and select a simillimum.

A young man aged 28 years who had complaint of vascular headache since year 2000 came to seek my treatment. His history revealed the following. Usually the pain begins in one eye mostly the left eye extends to left cranium and then to maxilla, mandible, nose left side, left side of neck and only occasionally shifting to right. He is also a known case of 'Chronic maxillary sinusitis.'

The pain apparently seemed to be a unilateral neuralgia and also sinusitis.

The pain is severe and he even feels pillow is pricking. The concomitants to the headache are a blocked nose, occasionally dark spots before the eyes, tickling in nose and profuse sweat on head. Increased thirst and irritability are the other concomitants. The headache is usually < From June to September[3+] every year < Sun[3+], Evening [2+]< drafts[3+], < Noise[3+], < light lying on painful side[3+] and< stooping , < change of weather[3] < , odours[3+]. > lying on abdomen[2+] are the other modalities. There is no associated vomiting or nausea . Blood pressure during the attacks is usually found to be 100/70 mm of hg pulse is normal. The complaints started after he had a sever attack of viral fever. Pains usually but only temporarily responds to Tab. Brufen. He is 5" ¾'" weight is 70 kg.

THE GENERALS

Appetite is good. Thirst[++] for chilled water.

Craves chilly food[3+] and rice[3+].

Spices lead to burning and bitter eructation.

Craves alcohol[2], Stools satisfactory, Urine h/o urine infection recently.

He gets profuse sweats on head otherwise and also during complaints.

He usually goes to sleep at 11.30 pm and gets up at 8.00 a m. The sleep is deep. He gets dreams of money[+++] and of his unfulfilled ambitions and occasionally startles in sleep. His Sexual desire is[++] and there is no history of indulgence, or contact.

Childhood reveals history of recurrent fever, chicken pox, worms, pica for lime.

Abdominal complaints, grinding of teeth jaundice once and typhoid twice.

One mole on neck and early graying of hair were found on physical examination.

INVESTIGATIONS

X-ray PNS Water's View.

Both maxillary sinuses show mucosal thickening, frontal sinuses NAD, No evidence of DNS Nasal fossa clear, Space is obliterated by hypertrophied turbinates.

Nasal endoscopy- WNL.

ENT opinion: Maxillary sinusitis with Rhinitis and Neuralgia

Family History:

Psora[2+], Sycosis[2+], Tubercle[2+].

LIFE SPACE

He has a very small friends circle he is basically reserved. He never talks on his own with others only if other people talk he talks. Never liked studies mediocre. Got 50% marks at Matriculation. Disliked mathematics always curious about electronic items. He presently deals in computer hardware, he has done his B.Com. Diploma in Electronics. Was happy when passed HSC examinations doesn't like mixing once he is angry over somebody never talks to him. Does share his problems with father with who he is attached [++]. Doesn't talk much at home, prefers to be alone. Doesn't like to go to social gatherings and ceremonies. Wants an independent house for himself he has desire for money[5+] but hesitates to ask for money even when it is due. If unable to attend calls of his customers he keeps thinking about it and that troubles him. He cannot easily forget and forgive. If gets into a fight he does express his anger strongly.

He feels sad of his inability to 'go ahead' in life, when he hears his friends going ahead in life. He gets a bad feeling when he sees any of his friends achieving something. He maintains good relations with clients and colleague. Sounds and talk often irritate him. He says he is not very resolved. Unable to implement his plans often lags behind time. At school he dislike study had a lot of anticipatory anxiety[3+] during exams. He hesitates to do daring on his own someone has to always force him to do things who may be his father or mother or brother. Says was frustrated when he did not get a job. The problematic clients produce a lot of anxiety and agitation and his performance before is affected. He is not much confident. Has a low self esteem. Lazy[3+] does not do shaving bathing, he is uncomfortable with new people. Bothers how he will behave in front of them. Shared things as a child. Says he is basically not irritable but has gone irritable due to his mental frustrations and disappointments. Presently money is everything for him money first and then values he concludes.

■

CHRONIC CASES

CASE 1

The parents of an eight year old child, studying in standard three approached the physician with prime complaint of recurrent worm infestation since the child was of two years age. Her presenting complaints were pain in abdomen, itching in anus < night[3+], excessive hunger, biting of teeth in sleep and excessive craving for sweets during. She is also susceptible to colds and recurrent attacks of tonsillitis, tonsils are enlarged and congested and she gets difficulty in deglutition usually < Winter[3+] < Change of season to wet[3+], Change of weather[2+]. She also complaints of recurrent aphthae without any peculiarities, except a dry mouth.

She has a thin built, whitish complexion and dark rings around her eyes. Her height is 4'3" (more for age) weight is 23 kg, normal. Thirst is moderate. She desires rice[3+] and is even found eating dry rice at times she also craves ice cream[3+], cold drinks[3+], green salads[3+]. She has h/o pica for earth[3] till 1 years age. The paediatrician had diagnosed calcium deficiency and disturbances in calcium metabolism then and calcium injections were given along with vitamin D. After which her pica was reduced. Her stools are satisfactory and once in the morning. Urine is normal H/o UTI at the age of 5 years. Her sweats are scanty and she sweats on head hands and feet. She has good sleep and sleeps for about 9 hours at night. She sees in her dreams that she has gone to a far away palace and playing with her friends. A flower has came to ear her, she is driving her mothers moped. Mothers gestation notes gives h/o nausea for first four months and aversion to milk. Mother was little tensed as her mother in law was ill and husband left the job. MIL died in 6th month of pregnancy. A USG opinion revealed that she had congenital polycystic kidneys. At one point of time a USG opinion expressed that the foetus may not be alive which was fortunately not true yet generated a   lot of anxiety in the parents.

All vaccinations were given at proper time responses to vaccination normal. Weaning 6-7th month accepted well birth wt 2.5 kg. normal delivery. Mile stones turning at 2½m, 4 –5th month, crawling 8th month. On her first birthday she spoke monosyllables and on the second birthday small sentences, she was standing with support in 14 to 16th month. Desires warm bath all through the year except summer but still wants luke warm water. She has desires for covers ++ summer light covers preferred, fanning. Wants less food as served.

Since 2½ years ages she slept less and was obviously hyperactive³⁺, talkative. She gets excited over little things and her father says she over reacts. She is a timid child, extremely sensitive, weepy over small things at her school, which disturb her and trouble her. She is deeply attached to her near relatives. If things become monotonus loss interest, she can not concentrate. Easily mixes, is careless, does share things, is shy with new people and doesn't talk with them. Even if mother and father are talking about some serious matter she starts to weep and is evidently anxious. She fears dog and darkness. Likes writing reading likes colours, cartoons, love stories, horror movies, fears class teacher, remembers past things but is absent minded and forgets recent occurrence. Her family history reveals strong tubercular trait. There are white spots on her three nails.

TOTALITY OF SYMPTOMS

Family History

Strong tubercular trait.

Past history

Poly-cystic disease.

Calcium absorption weakness of bones.

Desire for clay, earth till 2 years.

Otitis media thrice.

Mother mentally tensed during the pregnancy, anxiety[3+].

Till 5 years of age bed wetting.

Eruptions skin- hands, legs, left eye lid disappeared by homeopathic treatment (Graphites 30).

Milestones- turning at 2½ months (Normal is 3½ to 4 months).

Thermality

Chilly patient[5+].

Generals

Modalities < Change of weather to wet[3+].

< winter[3+].

Sensations

Mentals:

Intelligent.

Timid[3+]- Fear of darkness and dog.

Touchy[3+].

Weepy[3+].

Active[+].

Talkative[+].

Attached^{++}.

Shy.

Careless.

Restless.

Physical

Thin built whitish complexion 4 feet 3 inches more for her age.

Susceptible to colds^{3+}.

Biting of teeth during sleep and occasional talking during sleep.

Dreams fearful.

Craves Rice^{3+}, likes Dry rice^{3+}, Ice cream and Cold drinks^{3}+, sweets^{3+}, eats sugars, green salads^{2+3}.

Averse bitter gourd, spinach and coconut.

Characteristic particulars

Worm infestation since two years of age.

Biting of teeth during sleep.

Pain in abdomen.

Itching anus.

Location

GIT.

REMEDY SELECTION

A case well recorded is half cured. This particular case demonstrates how a well recorded case itself furnishes us the image of the remedy in this case Calcarea phos. 200 was the obvious choice. It is worthy to note that Calc. phos. was selected the remedy for this case not only because many features of Calc. and Phos. are covered by this case but the case also has the peculiar features; which characterize the remedy also characterize this patient.

The essence of the remedy and the patient thus resemble. Family history (tubercle) thermality further supports the selection of this tubercular remedy[3]. Besides the patient presents with mental and physical feature of both Calcarea and Phosphorus. Three doses of 200 potency were given in three months. The patient no more has worm trouble and shows general improvement also.

CASE 2

A lady aged 42 years, B. com and a housewife married at the age of 19 years strictly vegetarian has complaint of hair fall since ten years. She had honeybee poisoning (bites all over body including scalp) after that she developed dandruff according to her after that her complaints started aggravation. Since three years aggravated. She has deep cracks both soles $<$ winter^{3+} $<$ summer^{2+} since many years ago last two years. She also complaints of acidity $<$ chill^{3+} spicy^{2+}, oily food^{2+}. She gets sour eructations and hiccough. At least once in summer she has bleeding from nose. She has a stocky built, whitish complexion, hair on cheek, her height is 5'1". Appetite is good. Thirst $++$ $<$ evening, winter. She has craving for sour^{3+} h/o pica for coal, slate, pencils. Sleep is alert, refreshing around six hours. At night shudders, startled in sleep.

Dreams of dead snakes, fearful and anxious dreams, and of her religious guru backing her in trying situations.

Menstrual history FMP 15½ years. Cycles usually regular four day, flow $<$ at night clots $^{++}$. Weakness $^{++}$ before during and after menses irritable before menses. Leucorrhoea $<$ exertion^{3+} itching.

She was number three child amongst the siblings and stayed in joint family with plenty of relatives. Her father was post master general. She wanted to complete M. Com but was married and now feels she should have done it. Her overall academic performance is average and didn't have a good memory. She was not much ambitious, had four close friends two of them were rich and at one point of time she felt she should not continue her friendship with them.

After her marriage due to sudden death of her MIL she was suddenly burdened with family responsibilities. She was not confident about being able to successfully shoulder her responsibilities and was anxious too. She feels she is doing so much for others and has shouldered all responsibilities well, yet the god and other people often disappoint her. She blames god for that. Her son's failure at the HSC greatly disturbed her, she was in depression owing to that. She often gets the feeling 'she alone has to do everything. And nobody has the realization of that.' She fears accident. She took so much care of the son during the entire year looked after every minor thing yet her son failed. Her husband is busy and she often feels lonely. She is emotional-feels somebody should be there. Some times she feels why she is obeying all her responsibilities so devotedly when no one has got the realization. She has faith in a religious guru and does what ever well say.

All her anger is expressed on her. She has to keep balance. Says she doesn't keep in mind things for a much longer time. Personal things are last in her agenda. She doesn't express her anger even when she gets angry, feels that will spoil things, she gets sleepless on such days. As a student feared exams had a lot of anxiety before exams. She is basically social but after her son failed she doesn't like going to functions. Although a wife of a high court judge she has no false concepts of ego. These days cries over little things. She is close to everyone.

Normally she behaves in a manner that won't hurt others even a little, she anticipates in advance about the other person's thoughts and behaves accordingly. When she listens anybody speaking badly in spite of her good behaviour feels bad. She is loosing confidence, cannot take decisions.

Once a student from her class had died she didn't have the courage to get up and go to her home to bid adieu. She gets greatly anxious if her husband gets little late to reach home. She is timid yet likes horror movies. Fears small things, fears to be alone. She thinks of everyone but nobody thinks of her. Fears quarrels at home. Feels when she has done her job so honestly why is not god kind to her, why doesn't he give returns. Her thermals show that she is ambithermal towards chilly. Her family history reveals fundamental miasm as tubercle as also the presenting miasm.

TOTALITY OF SYMPTOMS

Family History
Fundamental miasm: Tubercular.

Past history
Typhoid.

Mental state
Intellect: Mediocre.

Memory poor.

Emotions: Anxiety, fear, sentimental.

Behaviour: Amiable, social.

Functioning: Responsible.

Thermality
Ambithermal towards cold[4+] (as per Boenninghausen's scale of thermality).

GENERALS

Sensations

Mental Evolution

Desires company

Fears to be alone, of accidents.

Attachment $^+$.

Expectations^{++} from people.

Unfulfilled expectations (no returns).

Disappointment^{3+}.

Anger^{3+}.

Fear of quarrels^{3+}.

Suppression of anger.

Vexation.

Outbursts on son.

Sadness.

Depressed.

Discouraged.

Lack of confidence.

Indecisive.

Withdrawn.

Seeks support of religious Guru.

Blames god.

Physical

Thirst $^{++}$ even in winter every hour.

Desires sour^3, spicy food^{2+}.

H/o Pica for coal, slate pencil.

Sweat $^{++}$.

Dreams of dead snakes of being supported by her guru in times of her tribulation.

Characteristic particulars

1. **Hair fall** ++ fifty to sixty hair per day.

   Hair growing thin.

   Dandruff $^+$, itching.

   Location: Scalp

2. **Modality:** < winter^{3+}.

   < summer.

   Sensation: Cracks, leg.

   Dry scales.

   Location: Skin soles.

3. **Modality:** < Chilly^{3+}.

   < spicy food^{3+}.

   < Oily food^{3+}.

   Sensation: Acidity^{++}.

   Eructation$^+$.

   Hiccough.

   Location: GIT.

4. **Modality:** < Night^{3+} (menstrual flow).

   < exertion (leucorrhoea).

   Sensation: Leucorrhoea.

   Irritable before menses.

   Pain in right hand.

   Clots$^+$.

   Modality: < Summer.

Sensation: Nose bleeding.

5.   **Hair on cheek**

Dark pigmentation neck.

REMEDY SELECTION

On the basis of above totality and with due considerations to the mentals of the patient Kali carb. was selected. Greater resemblance at the mental level pointed to the use of a higher potency, but pathological symptoms Hair fall and location skin pointed to the use of lower potency hence 30 potency was selected.

Treatment and follow up

10/12/04

Kali carb. 30 1p HS + Sac lac. 15 days.

25/12/04

No change Sac lac for 10 days.

Patient reported on 17/12/04 itching and dandruff less now, heartburns >/+.

Kali carb. 30 1p HS + SL for 15 days.

3/1/05

Hair fall less now, heartburns >2/+ SL for 20 days.

27/1/05

Hair fall less but continues little dandruff, no heartburns.

Kali carb. 30 1p HS + SL for 15 days.

7/2/05

Hair fall further reduced no dandruff or itching SL continued.

CASE 3

This is a case of a 51year old General surgeon suffering from Chronic tonsillo-pharyngitis, irritable bowel syndrome and acidity. This surgeon had a severe hospital staphylococal infection in 1974 and twice attacks of follicular tonsillitis since then developed susceptibility. O/E tonsil fibrosed and shrink, < cold water in summer^{3+}, <cold foods^{2+}, < exposure to cold^{3+}, there is sticky mucus in throat < 1 to 3 am night. He also has rhinitis of and on, < dust, summer < custard apple, using masks. He has frequent change of bowel habits colicky pain in abdomen < eating outer foods^{3+}, eating at unhygienic and even standard places, spicy food. There is h/o irregular food habits and hotel food for many years has to strain stools hard and soft, eating green leafy vegetables and high residue diet presently on Lactose and Chromaffin powder. Chronic dryness of hands and feet every time he washes his hands he has to apply moisturizer.

His height is 5'7", weight 65 kg appetite good, cravings for sweets^{3+} milk and milk products^{3+}, spicy food^{2+}. Averse to pumpkin and brinjal. Profuse urination at night. Sweats^{++} aggravation during sun, region on axilla. Sleeps at 10 pm and gets up at 6 am refreshing has to wake upto 3 times due to profuse urination. Dreams as everybody dreams I too dream he says, doesn't remember, dark children sitting on the top of a house on window.

Family history reveals a strong tubercular trait. Past h/o sensitivity to drugs, recurrent malaria, aphthous stomatitis, moles on body, neck^{1+}, face^{1+}, back^{1+}, extremities^{4+}. Allergic to detergents. O/E BP is N, pulse 68, nails corrugated, bilateral hernia, severe vascular headache.

The analysis and interpretation of the finding in the long life space of this patient revealed the following, which have been included in the totality of symptoms.

TOTALITY OF SYMPTOMS

Family history
Tubercular Miasm

Past history
Sensitive to Framycetin, Sulpha drugs, Cephalexin, Ciprofloxacin, Gentamycin.

Recurrent malaria 3-4 times.

Apthous stomatitis recurrent for 4-5 years.

Hernia right inguinal.

H/O Extreme sensitivity to cold.

Mental state
Intellect:	Intelligent[3+].
	Motivated.
	Conscientious.
Emotion:	Emotional/ Sentimental.
	Anger[3+] and Anxiety[3+].
Behaviour:	Excitable.
Functioning:	Uncompromising.
	Rebellious.

Thermality
Chilly Patient.

Generals
Modalities   - < Emotional stress[3+].

< Exposure to cold[3+].

SENSATIONS   (BOTH GENERALIZED MODALITIES)

General

Mentals

(Psychodynamics).

Ambitious.

Fastidious.

Egoist.

Attachment++.

Expectations from others and aspirations unfulfilled.

Sensitive.

Disappointment.

Vexation.

Brooder.

Irritable.

Hatred.

Jealous.

Agitational anxiety++.

Anticipatory anxiety++.

Fear.

Discouraged.

Sadness.

Wants salvation.

Physical

Craving for sweets[3+], spicy food[3+].

Childhood he used to kill ants and eat.

Sleep very alert, sleeplessness due to anxiety.

Dreams of his religious guru, 3-4 dark children sitting on the top of a house.

Characteristic Particulars

1. **Modality:** < Emotional stress^{3+}.

   < Exposure to cold^3.

   ⋌ Cold water, in summer^{3+}, or at night.

   < dust^{2+}.

   < custard apple.

   < 1to 3 am, Night (Mucous in throat).

   < Warmth^{2+}.

   Sensation: Irritation in throat.

   Mild pain during deglutition.

   Sneezing initially thin then yellow nasal. discharge.

   Sticky mucous in throat.

   Tonsils congested fibrosed and shrunken.

   Location: Upper respiratory tract.

2. **Modality:** < Eating foods^{3+}.

   < even eating at standard places^{2+}.

   < Spicy food.

   Sensation: Frequent change in bowel habits, constipation. weak urge to stool.

   Has to go 2 or 3 times unsatisfactory.

   Colicky pain in abdomen.

   Heartburn.

4. **Modality:** < Winter.

   Dryness of skin.

Every time he washes his hands with water he has to apply moisturizer.

REMEDY SELECTION

Natrum phos. 200 Potency was selected and in first three repetitions after 15 days, 1 month, one and half months gap the patient's bowel habits have been improved and he no more complaints of colicky pain and can endure hotel foods upto much extent. Nux vomica in 200 potency is the acute remedy. His treatment continues. Intercurrent remedy Tuberculinum 1M.

Features pointing to Tuberculinum strong tubercular history (P/H and F/H) Chilly^{5+} patient mentals intelligent^{3+}. Anger^{3+}, anxiety^{3+}, excitable, dissatisfaction. Skin dry susceptible to cold^{++} < emotional stress^{3+}, pathological findings- tonsils congested fibrosed shrunken.

CASE 5

A young girl, aged 26 years suffering from Bronchial asthma since the age of 13 years. She is susceptible to colds and usually has complaints of sneezing^{++}, < morning^{2+}, < evening^{3+}, thin discharge from nose which is usually followed by pharyngeal discomfort and a little burning in throat, slowly the cough with yellowish expectoration. Difficulty in respiration < exertion^{2+} < summer^{3+} < dry weather^{3+}, (recently), < smoke^{2+} < dust^{2+}, < wet getting^{2+}, < afternoon^{2+}, < sun^{2+}, < change of weather^{3+}, < lying down^{3+}, >head elevation^{2+}, < when anybody shouts^{3+}. There is history of < cold weather^{3+}, < rainy season^{3+} < after meal at night^{2+}, < cold drafts^{2+}, < cold fruits^{2+} ice cream, cold drinks. Fever, mild nose blockage, pain in occiput and forehead, thirst $^{++}$ every five minutes are the concomitants.

HISTORY OF PRESENT COMPLAINTS

At the age of 13 years one night she suddenly complained of pain in chest and severe difficulty in respiration so a local physician was consulted who advised some oral and injectable medicines to which she responded promptly in 2 three days. After that she started getting breathless on exertion and attacks of recurrent cold. Some two three years after the first attack she again had a severe attack but after that never had any attack.

Her associated complaints are headache[2+], occiput[2+], < talking[3+], < when shouted at[3+]. Pimples[++] all over the face suppurating –6 years < oily food, < summer[2+] .Motion sickness, nausea vomiting < traveling in bus < exposure to diesel fumes odour.

Patient as a person: General appearance- whitish complexion medium built weight 58 kg ht 5'4". Her appetite is[++] eats every 1-1½ hour when at home craves rice[2+], oily food[3+], sours[3+], spicy food[3+], junk food[3+], apple[2+], shrikhand[2+], aversion milk[3+]. Stools twice satisfactory. Sweats[3+] all over the body odour[+], stains [+]. Sleeps late wakes up late talks in sleep shouts at some one as if ailing dreams of murder[3+], fight[+], dreams of death[2+], with knife. Family history of sycosis, past history fall head injury.

Hb - 8.4 gm %, Anaemic

Menstrual History

FMP 15 years cycles regular 4days. h/o 1years only two days duration. Back ache before and during menses.

Thermals

Prefers cold water all through the year till march. Feels suffocated with hot water, covers less even in extreme winter[1+], thin cover. She desires fanning [++], season preferred is winter. She prefers warm food.

LIFE SPACE

She doesn't get along with any body. Mother says she is 'different' gets easily angered throws even costly thing in a fit of rage. She is angry < when ill. She failed in std 8 th due to complaints cried, cried and cried for many days after that she became irritable and obstinate till then she was silent studious girl. All childhood needs were met properly. She is jealous^{++} with her sibling. At SSC scored 49% and HSC scored 65%. Till sixth was good in studies after 7th here performance deteriorated says she cannot study as people at home trouble her. She doesn't do any household work and is lazy. She   doesn't do friendship with any one, lacks confidence, leaves things, courses incomplete, doesn't give her things to sibling if feels like talking, talks other wise doesn't talk. She doesn't talk with father who is angry back answers father. Likes watching TV, watches TV and sleeps for maximum period of the day. If anybody at home is talking in her reference she gets terribly angry. Prefers to be alone doesn't like to talk to anybody. Feels she is always right. She is anxious. Makes unreasonable demands from parents. She beats siblings. She is reserved^{3+}, lacks confidence^{3+}, possessive^{3+}, selfish^{3+}, lazy^{3+}, excitable arrogant^{3+}, dissatisfied jealous $^{++}$, dull desires^{++}, brooder indolent, indifferent.

TOTALITY OF SYMPTOMS

Family History

Sycosis

Past History

Measles and piles in childhood.

Fall injury to head.

Mental State

Intellect- Average.

Emotions- Anger^{3+}

Behaviour-Excitable.

Functioning- Indolent.

Thermality

Hot patient.

Generals

Modalities- < Summer^{3+}.

< Change of weather^{3+}.

< Wet getting^{3+}.

(Generalized in given case).

Sensations

Mental Evolution.

Desires $^{++}$.

Disappointment^{3+} (Because Average^{+} Indolent = Failure)

Brooder^{3+}.

Dissatisfaction^{+}.

Irritable^{3+}.

Sensitive takes easy offence.

Jealous $^{++}$.

Possessive.

Demanding.

Anxiety^{++}.

Lack of confidence.

Withdrawn.

Indifferent.

Physical

Susceptible to Colds^{3+}.

Anaemic, Hb 8.4gm%.

Thirst^{++}, wants water every 5 minutes.

Appetite^{++}, eats every hour.

Cravings oily food3, sour^{3+}, sweets^{2+} shrikhand^{2+}.

Aversion milk^{2+}

Sweats^{++}, odour offensive.

Sleeps late gets up late.

Shouts in sleep, as if fighting with someone.

Dreams of Murder^{3+}, fights^{2+}, death^{2+}.

Characteristic Particulars

Modality: < when anybody shouts at her^{3+}

   < Summer^{3+}

   < Change of weather^{3+}

· < wet getting^{3+}

   < Dry weather^{3+} (recently)

   < morning^{3+} (Cough and dyspnoea)

   < evening^{3+} (Sneezing)

   < lying down^{3+}

   < cold drafts^{2+}

   < Cold fruits, foods and drinks^{2+}

   < Exertion^{2+}

   < afternoon^{2+} (cough and dyspnoea)

   < smoke^{2+}

   < dust^{2+}

   < head elevation^{2+}

There is history of < cold weather^{3+}, < rainy season^{3+}.

Sensation:

Sneezing^{++} thin discharge from nose, which is usually followed by pharyngeal discomfort and a little burning in throat slowly the cough with yellowish expectoration. Difficulty in respiration.

   Concomitant: Fever, mild nose blockage, Pain in occiput and forehead, thirst $^{++}$ every five minutes are the concomitants.

   Location: Respiratory system.

2.   **Modality:** < When shouted at^{3+}

             < Talking.
     Sensation: Throbbing pain.
     Location: Head occiput.

3.   Since 5- 6 years.
     Pimples^{++}.
     Suppuration yellow.

4.   < Travel in bus and car^{3+}
     < Diesel odor^{3+}
     Nausea, vomiting.
     Severe backache $^{3+}$, before menses.

REMEDY SELECTION

   Strong family history of sycosis, a hot patient, resemblance at mental level, to the Natrum mind and similarity at the level of generals esp., modalities as well the as the characteristic particulars pointed to Natrum sulph. which was administered in 30 potency single dose was given to the patient to be taken at bed time after which the patient reported amelioration in her complaints.

   In the third follow up she was given the acute remedy Ars. iod. 30 one dose as the acute totality pointed to the remedy. Unfortunately the patient hasn't turned up after that.

ACUTE CASES

CASE 1

I had a case of gastroenteritis where there was a history of eating hotel foods and violent vomiting with severe pain around umbilicus. There were no modalities available in the case. I first prescribed Arsenic album 200 on the basis of the cause but it did not offer the relief. Next I prescribed Nux vomica 200 which too miserably failed. Then when the patient was in a state of collapse and agony too and I was thinking of referring him to the Government hospital, at this time father suddenly said 'Doctor do something for her stomachache, *if his stomach gets well, his vomiting will stop all his troubles lie in his stomach, in his umbilicus'* As many remedies were doing rounds to my mind like Veratrum album, Carbo veg. the illiterate father of the patient gave me the intelligent clue to the remedy telling me that everything else is insignificant in the case except a 'Sever umbilical colic' I prescribed Colocynth 200 and after a few frequent repetitions the patient was totally relieved of his sufferings.

So we must locate and treat root of suffering.

CASE 2

In a case of an old lady with generalized body pains without any modalities there were no characteristics available and there was just maze of multiple common symptom like backache, head ache, chest pain. I first prescribed remedies like Bryonia and Rhus tox which hardly helped. A little later I realized that the root of the suffering in the patient was in the flatulent stomach. The flatulence was everything that was destabilizing the economy and needed a remedy. This logic helped me to prescribe Carbo veg., which relieved her in a day. Such observations and logics do help us to become good prescribers.

CASE 3

This is a case that came to my elder brother, also a homoeopath, to him a middle aged lady came with complaint of agonizing pain in abdomen markedly aggravated by rest and lying down and characteristically ameliorated by motion. The restlessness and anxiety were also marked in the patient. In this case without giving due importance to the location Rhus tox was selected as its general picture resembled the general picture of the patient. A two hourly repetition of 200 potency the pain was relieve in a few hours.

CASE 4

In a case of Urticaria that occurred during a sudden change of weather to a damp coldness the itching was aggravated by covers and ameliorated by cold fomentation and uncovering. I prescribe Dulcamara 30 one dose taking into consideration the symptoms picture. Dulcamara failed to offer relief even after two days, the remedy was highly indicated considering the cause and modalities.

But soon I discovered that here more characteristic was that the urticaria although caused by a cold damp weather was aggravated by warmth and covers was ameliorate by washing with cold water. This characteristic contraindication lead to prescription of Pulsatilla a single dose of which worked wonders.

This case taught me to locate 'That' in a case on which the prescription should be based. This 'that' is the highly characteristic symptom or the 'highly valuable thing or a point' in a case which needed to be identified. It was a typical case of 'mistaken identity'

CASE 5

A three year old child came to me, with acute coryza and cough since one day, the previous night the cough[++] < lying down. The discharge from nose was thin irritating, expectoration was yellowish green. The generals were Appetite[++], Thirst[+], for little quantity frequently. Aversion to covers, hot patient. H/o usually respiratory complaints < winter[3], Arsenic Iod was selected in this particular case a single dose of 30 potency promptly offered the relief. Here patient's generals (esp. Aversion to covers, with characteristic Arsenicum thirst and Iodum appetite) together with characteristic particulars (which resemble the remedy) lead to this prescription.

CASE 6

A middle-aged man came to me with h/o itching wheels on legs only around the knees. The itching was severe and led to burning. There was a history of application of Ayurvedic ointment and use of new kneecap. He had recently started with internal allopathic medication of an orthopedic surgeon for his rheumatic trouble. There was a history of allergy to allopathic drugs especially Paracetamol and Nimesulide, surprisingly this time the orthopaedician's prescription did not include these drugs. Suspecting hypersensitivity reaction to either of the three things- Ayurvedic ointment, allopathic drugs and new knee cap, Nux vomica 200 two doses were given one on the night when the patient approached this physician and another the next morning. There was a marked amelioration on the next day evening, on the third day the eruptions disappeared. Here again locating the cause led to the correct prescription.

CASE 7

A case of heat exhaustion came to me in mid summer. The symptoms were extreme weakness, tremors, headache esp. occiput and palpitation. The blood pressure was 100/70 mm of hg the pulse was 90/min. Thirst was normal, moderate. On the so demonstrable picture Gelsemium 200 repeated three hourly brought the patient back to normal.

CASE 8

A thirty year old man came to me with dark, small spots on extremities with scratch marks and scars due to injury from scratching. According to him the eruptions were very itchy and red initially but turned dark on scratching. Itching always led to severe burning. A further inquiry reveled that they appeared on the next day after he ate mutton the previous Sunday, he rarely eat mutton and usually preferred chicken on the weekends.

The cause of eating meat and typical features of the scar lead to the simple selection of Arsenic album 30 the single dose of which was given and eruptions disappeared in 5 days.

CASE 9

An old lady had loose motions four to five times after the news of the death of her nephew. Her thirst was[++] and she had little tremors, per abdomen examination revealed nothing. There were no other symptoms in the case. Here Ignatia 200 repeated three hourly relieved her and also stabilized her. Here too preference to the cause led to the correct prescription.

CASE 10

A young lady who had given birth to a female child just two months back came with complaints of red itching spots on fore arms and face especially maxilla for last fifteen days. There was no h/o urticaria or any drug allergy. There were no modalities in the case neither marked generals. As I was thinking 'what to prescribe?' The patient just remarked that usually the spots itch more after she comes back home from market or any other outing. It was the month of April. Then I made and inquiry into how long did she go out in sun for the first time after the delivery. According to her it was almost a month and a half she went out in sun because of the Post-partum restrictions by parents. I logically concluded that the eruptions were nothing but sunburns. The causation and modality lead to the prescription of Canth. 30 two doses were repeated after the gap of four days. In ten days the complaints were completely relieved.

CASE 11

A case of right sided menstrual colic > warm formentation[3+] and pressure[2+].

Appetite diminished thirst normal restlessness due to pain in a chilly patient with irritability during menses. In this case Mag phos. 200 'did the honours'.

CASE 12

A 20 year old man came to me with boils on back and forearms, without itching, no pus, only little pain. The only cause ascertained was perspiration as he worked near furnace. With Rhus tox 30 one dose, the eruptions disappeared in seven days.

F - 13

CASE 13

A house wife came with a catch in the back spasmodic pain < motion^{3+} < getting up^{3+}, <after prolonged sitting^{3+} amelioration lying down. H/O sleeping on cold floor. I was a little confused over the selection of the drug as some modalities pointed to Bryonia and some to Rhus tox but giving due importance to the probable cause and few modalities Rhus tox 200 was repeated four hourly which totally relieved the patient.

CASE 14

An old widow aged 66 years came to me one fine morning. In the waiting hall she almost dropped herself on the bench and had to be brought inside by the attendants at my clinic. The picture suggested a 'Critical' condition. On examination her blood pressure was found to be 106/70 mm of Hg, her pulse was 60 per minute. The systemic examination revealed nothing. She was afebrile. She complained of extreme weakness and palpitation and soon it was clear that it was rather a case of acute anxiety attack than anything else. She said that she was feeling tremendously week and became anxious as soon she came to know that soon she had to stay all alone since her only grandson staying with her was leaving the city for another job. She was also feeling chilly. Many remedies like Gelsemium, Argentum Nitricum came to my mind Arsenic Album was selected since Anxiety^{++} and weakness out of proportion of the ailments and chills characteristically pointed to it. Few doses of 200 potency made the patient much better in a day.

CASE 15

In A young lady who took the treatment of a Gynaecologist to delay her menstrual date owing to a religious programme at home a few months back the menses had not returned even after three months. She didn't have any complaints at all. Normally she had a 28 day cycle, with duration of 4-5 days. Discharge- bright red blood, no clots no complaints before during and after the menses. LMP was 03/09/04 and EMP, which was delayed by allopathic medication was 30/10/04. What to prescribe in such a case was a difficult question.

I prescribed Nux vomica 200 three doses at bed time on three consecutive day. The menses appeared within a week. The only thing that was aimed in this case without any symptoms was to 'Remove the bad effects of patent medicine'.

CASE 16

A middle-aged man came to me with history of profuse diarrhoea and severe vomiting since one day. He had neglected his complaints for a day. Drinking even a little water induced vomiting, there was also a history of eating food outside. He looked extremely pale, weak and dehydrated. The skin was cold to touch. The blood pressure was found to be 100/66 mm of hg and pulse 96/min. Thirst+ was for normal water. He had cramps in calves. I was about to prescribe Arsenic album on the basis of his complaints when I realized that in the case more than anything the importance should be given to the 'pale collapsed type' picture of patient together with a cold skin and cramp in calves and I selected Veratrum album a few doses in 1M potency offered prompt relief. Here the 'Picture of the Patient' resembled more to Veratrum Album than Arsenic album which is noteworthy.

CASE 17

A six month old child came to me with history of thin discharge per nose and dry cough since two days. There were no other things that characterized the case. I was hesitant to prescribe a remedy to this infant considering his age and paucity of symptoms. It was a rainy weather. A month back I had prescribed the same patient Rhus tox 30 one dose for his milk rash. Rhus tox being the only remedy found safe since earlier administered to him by me and supported by the weather was prescribed which cured his cough and coryza in three days.

CASE 18

As this particular case suggests some times chronic remedies may be prescribed in acute cases if the characteristic picture of the ailment resembles the remedy in a particular sector. In a seven year old child who had cough since 22 days with white expectoration and wheezing typically aggravated between 2 to 4 am with vomiting on coughing, the patient being chilly. At last I prescribed Kali carb 30 single dose which relieved him promptly. My previous prescriptions failed to relieve since they weren't as close to him as Kali carb. In rare cases deep acting chronic remedies may be used in minimum doses if the acute picture points to them. They should be avoided where pathological changes have set in. Yet injudicious use of chronic remedies for acute ailments must be avoided.

CASE 19

A case of burning per rectum in a patient with silent piles severely aggravated due to homoeopathic treatment without any history of bleeding. Nux vom. 30 as an antidote offered relief in one dose. Here it is important to note that the patient being drugged by homeopathic medicine potency in lower range was used.

CASE 20

One of my patient on chemotherapy for breast cancer, off and on complained of burning in epigastrium and had attacks of loose motions and violent vomitings. She always responded to Nux vomica in 200 potency. It just happened once that this physician without going into details of the case prescribed the 'usual remedy' Nux vomica and this time the patient didn't respond to it because although the cause and the nature of complains were the same, the generals of the patient which were observed later, i. e. rapid extreme weakness and thirst for little quantity frequently and anxiety belonged to Arsenic album which was the right remedy.

CASE 29

BIBLIOGRAPHY

Samuel Hahnemann: *Organon of medicine* 5th and 6th edition, *Chronic diseases, Hahnemann's lesser writings.*

M. L. Dhawale: *Principles and Practice of Homeopathy.*

Clinical investigation in Homeopathic practice, The ICR operational manual.

J. T. Kent: *Lesser writings.*
Lectures on Homeopathic philosophy,
Lectures on Homeopathic Materia medica.
Repertory of Homeopathic Materia Medica

Stuart Close: *Genius of homeopathy.*

H.A. Roberts: *The art of cure by homeopathy.*

Von Boenninghuasen: *Therapuetic Pocket Book.*